NOT YET PREGNANT

NOT YET PREGNANT

Infertile Couples in Contemporary America

ARTHUR L. GREIL

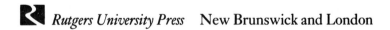 *Rutgers University Press*   New Brunswick and London

To Barbara, who waited with me,
and to Robby, who was worth waiting for

———————

Some material in this book has been previously published in different forms: "Infertility: His and Hers," co-authored with T. A. Leitko and K. L. Porter, *Gender & Society* 2 (1988):172–199 (copyright 1988 by Sage Publications, Inc.); "Couple Infertility as a Social Disability," in *Advances in Medical Sociology*, volume 2, edited by Gary A. Albrecht and Judith A. Levy (Greenwich, Conn.: JAI Press, 1991); "Technology of Reproduction: Religious Responses," *The Christian Century* 106 (1989):11–14 (copyright 1988 by The Christian Century Foundation); "Sex and Intimacy among Infertile Couples," co-authored with T. A. Leitko and K. L. Porter, *Journal of Psychology and Human Sexuality* 11 (1989):117–138; "Why Me?: Theodicies of Infertile Men and Women," co-authored with K. L. Porter, T. A. Leitko, and C. Riscilli, *Sociology of Health and Illness* 11 (1989):213–229 (reprinted with permission of Basil Blackwell Ltd.). I am grateful to the publishers for their kind permission to reprint.

Library of Congress Cataloging-in-Publication Data

Greil, Arthur L.
   Not yet pregnant : infertile couples in contemporary America /
Arthur L. Greil.
      p.   cm.
   Includes bibliographical references and index.
   ISBN 0-8135-1682-X (cloth) — ISBN 0-8135-1683-8 (pbk.)
   1. Marriage—United States.   2. Childlessness—United States.
3. Infertility—Social aspects—United States.   4. Infertility—
United States—Psychological aspects.   I. Title.
HQ734.G743   1991
306.872—dc20   90-21142
                                                                                       CIP

British Cataloging-in-Publication information available

CONTENTS

v

ACKNOWLEDGMENTS

My name is the only one that appears on the cover, but this book could not have been written without the help of many others. First and foremost, I thank the infertile wives and husbands I interviewed. These people allowed me to come into their homes because they believed that my book would help other infertile couples. Now that they see the final product of our collective effort, I hope they feel that their faith in me was justified.

My ideas about infertility and its social context have been influenced over the years by conversations I have had with Ellen Asprooth, Barbara Greil, Mark Jackson, Judith N. Lasker, and Barbara Katz Rothman. Thomas A. Leitko was intimately involved with this project in its early stages, and, although his participation ended several years ago, the final product has clearly benefited from his collaboration. Karen L. Porter was willing to step in on short notice to help me complete the interviewing process; since that time, she has remained a supportive colleague and an insightful critic.

Both the Alfred University Summer Grant Program and the Scholarly Activities Committee of the College of Liberal Arts and Sciences provided me with much-needed funding. I received able research assistance from Karen Leschinski, Patricia Nowetner, Catherine Riscilli, and Scott Schermerhorn. Barbara Scranton spent many hours typing transcripts. Thomas Conlon, Karen Mix, and Cheryl Monroe provided assistance with the typing of various versions of the manuscript. Barbara Greil, Pam Lakin, Frank McBride, and Lana Meissner helped with literature searches. Linda Hardy and Trevor Jones always made an effort to find promptly the interlibrary loan materials I ordered.

Alfred University funded my sabbatical leave during the 1989–1990 academic year, when I completed the bulk of the writing. I spent my sabbatical year as a research associate in Women's Studies at the University of Pittsburgh. I am grateful to the Women's Studies Program for providing me with the opportunity to do research at Pitt and making me feel welcome. Lynn Davidman, Jonathan Ehrlen, Irene Frieze, Carol McAllister, and Daniel Regan were especially instrumental in making my year in Pittsburgh enjoyable and productive.

Lynn Davidman, Judith N. Lasker, and Catherine Kohler Riessman read the entire manuscript carefully. Their insightful comments and suggestions have been of tremendous help to me. I would also like to thank Judith Lorber, Barbara Katz Rothman, and a score of anonymous reviewers whose comments on various articles I have written on the subject of infertility have helped shape many ideas I express in this book.

It has been a delight to work with Marlie Wasserman, my editor at Rutgers University Press. She has been supportive and helpful throughout what has turned out to be a relatively painless process.

My wife, Barbara Greil, has been a constant source of encouragement throughout the period of research and writing. My son, Robby, has been very patient and considerate during what must have seemed to him like a very long time.

ONE

INTRODUCTION
The Social Construction of Infertility

L iz, an elementary school teacher, and Matt, a manager in a state agency, had been married about eight years when I interviewed them. Liz and Matt had not seen having children as a high priority when they first married, but it did not take too long for them to change their minds. Liz thought they started to try to conceive about a year after their marriage; Matt thought it might have been somewhat longer.

After about a year of "trying," Liz began to suspect that something might be wrong and consulted her regular gynecologist. After "running the regular tests," including an x-ray called a hysterosalpingogram, Dr. Nathan thought he detected some hormonal irregularities and put Liz on a common infertility drug called clomiphene citrate. She became pregnant the next month.

Three months later, Liz had a miscarriage. Following the miscarriage, she found that she was unable to become pregnant again. On Liz's initiative, she and Matt started going to an infertility specialist at a major medical center in a city about seventy-five miles from their home. Liz took a leadership role throughout the infertility treatment process. As Matt put it, "She tends to be the spark plug in this operation."

After several different drug therapies failed to achieve the desired results, Liz asked Dr. Wolcott to do another hysterosalpingogram. He did so and discovered that the first x-ray had been misread. Liz's tubes were both blocked. All the hormones in the world weren't going to help if the tubes were not repaired. Liz still doesn't understand how she was able to become pregnant the first time.

Over the next five years, Liz had seven tubal surgeries, all unsuccessful. In addition, she spent many months on Human Menopausal Gonadotropin (hMG), a drug often used to stimulate ovulation when clomiphene citrate has proven ineffective. While she was on hMG, Liz had to make frequent seventy-five-mile trips to get shots. Matt estimates the costs of these treatments at $45,000.

Liz found the experience of infertility devastating. Everywhere she went, she encountered reminders of her inability to become pregnant. She thought constantly about why this was happening to her, but she was unable to come up with a satisfying answer. She describes her reaction to her infertility:

> I was so sad, and I couldn't figure out how to get happy. I mean I looked at all those people around, and everybody could get pregnant but me. And especially working, teaching. I'd see all these families that didn't take care of their kids and that had eight, or nine, or ten, and they were dirty, and they weren't dressed. Then it became almost an anger with God and me. I wasn't a good churchgoer, but all along I just kept praying and praying. Then, when I never got pregnant, I really became angry with God because if there was a God, you know, how could that happen? Well, it was unfair, and God wasn't to me quite fair.

In an effort to escape from reminders of her infertility, Liz pulled away from several of her fertile friends. At one point, she seriously considered going back to school to prepare herself for a career where she would not deal with small children.

Liz was frustrated by the lack of success they were having with treatment, but she couldn't bring herself to stop trying. She recounted:

> We'd set deadlines. "If we're not pregnant by Christmas, then we'll stop." Well, then Christmas would come, and I wasn't pregnant, so then what? So then we'd say, "Well, okay, we'll try one more surgery and see what happens." And, every time, nothing would happen. I don't know how we would ever have stopped if we hadn't adopted Ryan. It was terribly frustrating because I couldn't seem to stop doing it. It was just compulsive because we wanted a baby.

Matt saw infertility as a disappointment but not a tragedy. It was just one of those things people go through: "I have a good life. I see myself as having a good life, and I'm glad of that. I'm glad that I do have a nice life here and I always kind of try to take the philosophy of, you know, look at how bad that guy's got it." Matt took the attitude that it was always best to look on the bright side of things. Although he was concerned about their infertility, he was able to find satisfaction in his hobbies and other aspects of his life. Liz said: "He would have stopped treatment before I would have. But he had other things. He had a lot of hobbies, and I just wanted to be a mother." As Liz related, she was not always comforted by Matt's stoic acceptance of their infertility: "I was angry at him because I didn't think it really affected him like it did me, and that made me angry. I just felt that his life was good and my life wasn't." For his part, Matt thought Liz was overreacting. He felt that she should try to make more of an effort to put infertility behind her so that they could get on with their lives.

But in spite of both their different responses to infertility and the tension it introduced into their relationship, Liz and Matt feel that the experience of infertility has strengthened rather than weakened their relationship. According to Liz, "I think it made us closer because we had a common problem. We were trying to achieve the goal of having a child, and, for one reason or another, we couldn't. So, in order to solve the problem, we had to pull together."

Matt and Liz had adopted their son, Ryan, about a year before I interviewed them, after deciding that they had just about run out of viable medical options. According to Liz, adopting Ryan has made a big difference in her outlook on life:

> I don't know how I would have held up religiously if infertility had just gone on and on without a child or else at least a new job that really satisfied me. I mean, I don't think I could have just accepted infertility without having some resolution either child-wise or job-wise come out of it that was positive and still have faith because I was getting quite upset with that. But because things did work out, it's hard for me to talk about infertility as infertility because infertility, at this point in our lives, is what led up to Ryan. And I look at him, and I feel that it was all kind of meant to be, I guess.

SOME QUESTIONS

Liz and Matt are not fictional, nor do they form a composite of all the infertile couples I interviewed. They are real. I have given them pseudonyms, but I have not changed any details of their stories. I have not put any words into their mouths; rather, I have quoted them verbatim. Because they are real, they are not absolutely typical of the at least 2.4 million infertile couples in the United States or even of the ones I spoke to. Every infertile couple is unique; each has its own story to tell.

But in many ways, Liz and Matt *are* typical. Liz, like many other infertile wives, found the experience of infertility all-consuming and devastating, something she could not put behind her. Matt, like many other infertile husbands, saw infertility as a bad break, not a tragedy. Like many other infertile couples, Liz and Matt found that their different responses to infertility led to tension in their marriage.

4

But, also like most other infertile couples, Liz and Matt weathered the storm; Matt even sees infertility as bringing them closer together.

Like many other infertile wives, Liz found herself "addicted" to treatment, willing to go to almost any lengths to achieve her goal of having a baby. And like many other infertile wives, Liz experienced infertility, not just as a medical crisis but also as a threat to meaning and a challenge to her faith.

In this book I try to describe and explain the ways in which contemporary American couples experience infertility. I attempt to answer several questions:

Why do women and men respond so differently to infertility? What are the consequences of gender differences in the experience of infertility?

How have changes in medical technology changed the experience of infertility?

Why is it so difficult for infertile couples, especially infertile wives, to make sense out of the experience of infertility?

Why are infertile couples, especially infertile wives, so committed to pursuing the goal of bearing children?

This last question is perhaps the most fascinating and most important to our discussion.

INFERTILITY IN SOCIAL CONTEXT

Implicit in the questions I have just raised is the viewpoint that infertility is not merely a physiological condition and that the experience of infertility is not determined by the physiological fact of infertility itself. Sociologists Joseph Schneider and Peter Conrad have recently argued that medical sociologists ought to develop an "ethnography of

illness" that focuses on the ways in which people who define themselves as ill and who are defined as ill experience illness.[1] The same
argument can be made for infertility.

I think it is useful to distinguish between infertility as a medically
diagnosed physiological characteristic of individuals, which I call *reproductive impairment*, and infertility as a socially constructed reality
experienced by couples. The existence of a physiological impairment in one or both partners does not in and of itself determine the
course of couples' experiences of infertility. Rather, the process of
being infertile is dialectical; husbands and wives interpret, respond
to, and give meaning to physical symptoms and physiological conditions. Diagnoses and recommendations for treatment provided by
physicians help shape couples' interpretations of their infertility, but
they do not dictate the nature of husbands' and wives' interpretations. Husbands and wives may disbelieve physicians' interpretations, they may add their own interpretations to physicians' versions
of their experiences, or they may try to manage information so as
to influence physicians' diagnoses. The most important decisions
couples make as they define and resolve their crises of infertility—
whether to seek treatment, whether to undergo a particular diagnostic test, whether to stop treatment, whether to pursue adoption,
whether to explore *in vitro* fertilization (IVF), and so on—are not
medical decisions at all.

The rule of thumb commonly employed by medical professionals
is that a couple is considered infertile if the wife has not conceived
after twelve months of unprotected intercourse or if either partner
has a known condition that makes conception unlikely. Socially and
psychologically, however, couples without documented medical
problems can feel infertile even if they have not tried to conceive for
the twelve-month period indicated by the medical definition. Such
couples, though not infertile by the medical definition, may still experience the same thoughts, emotions, and self-definitions as couples
who are reproductively impaired. Conversely, couples with documented or documentable reproductive problems may not endure the
social experience of infertility. For example, a woman who does not

ovulate but who does not desire children may think of herself not as infertile but as voluntarily childless.

From a social construction perspective, infertility is not to be viewed as a static *condition* with psychosocial consequences, but as a dynamic, socially conditioned *process* whereby couples come to define their inability to bear their desired number of children as problematic and attempt to interpret and correct this situation.

Because each couple is unique, that couple's experience of infertility is unique. But this is not to say that each infertile couple fashions a response to infertility out of whole cloth. A couple's experience of infertility is shaped by the ideology and social structure of the society in which they live. It is influenced, among other things, by the nature of medical technology in a given society, by the functions of marriage and the family in that society, by role expectations for men and women, and by the social value of children. It is also influenced by beliefs about the importance or nonimportance of blood relationships, by ideas about the relative contributions of men and women to the processes of conception and child rearing, by general theories about the causes and cures of health problems, by societal beliefs about the nature of moral action and the causes of suffering, and so forth.

INFERTILITY AND CULTURAL VARIABILITY

Perhaps the most dramatic way to make the case that the experience of infertility is socially constructed is to look briefly at some varied beliefs and practices associated with it, ideas that exist and have existed in various cultures throughout the world. To simplify matters, I focus here on primary infertility, involuntary childlessness.

First, not all cultures share the same definition of what it means to be childless. In traditional Korea and Taiwan, where a son was required to perform ancestor rituals and to insure family continuity, having no sons had virtually the same practical consequences as being childless. [2]

Cultures differ in the extent to which they attribute importance to blood relationships, and this almost certainly affects both how infertility is regarded and what is done about it. While Korea and Taiwan both emphasized the importance of sons, the traditional cultural responses to the lack of sons have been quite different in the two societies. In Korea, where adopted children were regarded as full family members, one could solve the problem by adopting a son. But in Taiwan, where blood ties have been culturally more important, the traditional response to having no sons has been to adopt a *daughter* in the belief that doing so would "call in a younger brother." In some cultures, such as the African Hausa, the Iban of Borneo, and the Objibwa Indians, adoption has been so common that almost half, and sometimes over half, of all households included adopted children.[3] The experience of infertility in such societies almost inevitably differs from societies where blood ties are held paramount.

Societies differ with regard to the roles open to women. In many traditional societies women have virtually no alternatives to the domestic roles of wife and mother. Anthropologists Paul and Laura Bohannon write that, among the Tiv of Nigeria, a woman's total social role depends on having children because her place in this patrilineal society stems from being the mother of a lineage member. In many societies, men whose wives have borne no children may legitimately divorce them. An ethnographer who told his Dogon informant that he had no children was solemnly instructed that he must divorce his wife and marry again. In a number of cultures, including the East African Ganda, the Middle Eastern Kurds, and the Tucano of South America, a man whose wife has had no children may take a second wife.[4] One comparative study found this to occur in thirty-one of the forty-two societies for which adequate data could be found.[5] It seems likely that the precariousness of the social situation of childless women in the cultures we have been describing will have an impact on their experience of infertility.[6]

In many cultural groups, including Greek and Polish peasants, Oceanic Truk islanders, and Klamath Indians, infertility has been regarded as exclusively a physical problem for the wife. On the other hand, the Ashanti believe that only men can be infertile. Still other groups, such as the Oceanic Tikopia, the Hopi, and the South American Amayra have acknowledged that infertility could be due to either male or female reproductive impairments.[7] Such cultural beliefs about who is susceptible to infertility almost certainly influence the experience of infertility.

Infertility has been attributed to many causes, some physiological, some supernatural. The Ganda believe that infertility occurs when a woman's womb has turned over. The Dogon and the Ashanti say that infertility sometimes results from difficulties in the marital relationship. According to the Trukese, the hard work that women do may lead to a "bad stomach," which causes infertility. The Amhara believe that women's infertility follows from "loose living."[8]

The North African Somali attribute infertility to astrological influences. The Toradja of the Central Celebes Islands consider that infertility may be the result of the ancestors' anger at an oversight in the performance of a couple's marriage ritual; they attempt to rectify the situation by resanctifying the marriage. For the Ashanti, the source of the problem is usually a witch who has eaten the spiritual counterpart of a woman's womb or a man's penis. The Ndembu of Zambia generally ascribe a woman's infertility to the fact that she has been "caught" by the shade of a recently deceased ancestor. The Pawnee held that infertility could be induced by breaking cultural taboos concerning pubic hair. Polish peasants attribute infertility to God's will.[9]

Most societies do not attribute infertility to a single cause. Among the Bemba, infertility may be attributed to a curse on the part of the father's sister, to an injured spirit returning to punish a descendant at random, to allowing the umbilical cord of a baby to fall to the ground, to adultery, or to witchcraft. Spirit mediums of the Aowin people of Ghana may diagnose infertility as caused by witchcraft, nonobservance of prescribed behavior, disrupted social relationships, or quarrels between matrilineal kin.[10]

Just as cultures vary widely with regard to their beliefs about the causes of infertility, so too do they vary with regard to their ideas about what is to be done about it. Solutions open to the traditional Taiwanese peasant woman included appealing to the gods, consulting a diviner who could read her "flower fortune," trying herbal remedies, and adopting a female child to encourage the birth of a son. A visitor among the Dogon who admitted he was childless was asked if he had tried the following remedies: Had he prayed to God? Had he taken herbal medicines prepared by a diviner? Had he sacrificed at his father's altar? Had he looked for a second wife? Had he asked a brother or a friend to give him a child? Cultures vary with regard to the degree to which adoption solves the problem of infertility. For example, on Truk, a childless woman will commonly request a child of her sister or brother, and apparently she is rarely refused. Among the Toradja, a childless couple has the *right* to adopt a kin group member.[11]

Because almost all my examples are from preindustrial societies, it may seem that the case I am trying to make for the experience of infertility, as culturally and socially constructed, may be valid for such societies but less relevant to our own society, where popular understandings of infertility are informed by the perspective of modern, scientific medicine. I argue, however, that the notion of socially constructed infertility can be usefully applied to all societies.

First, we must be careful not to assume that the world views of ordinary people in contemporary society are always based on scientific logic and scientific evidence. Many Americans share some beliefs about infertility that are not much different from views common in less complex societies. Like Taiwanese peasants, many Americans believe that adopting a child will bring on a biological child. Like Truk islanders and Klamath Indians, many Americans see infertility as exclusively a women's problem. Many who recognize that men, too, can be infertile associate male infertility with impotence. While Americans seldom advise their infertile friends to visit a sacred shrine, the often-heard recommendation to take a vacation may perhaps be regarded as a secularized version of the same solution.

Second, we must not be so quick to equate the medical with the scientific. The shape taken by medical institutions in our society—or in any other—is by no means simply determined by scientific necessity. Psychiatrist Howard Stein has recently pointed out that medicine itself can be understood as a subculture with shared understandings about what constitutes moral action, the proper role of patients, the value of money, and so on. Journalist Lynn Payer has shown that, among the developed societies of the West, notions of what constitutes proper medical practice vary considerably from one society to the next. Medical understandings, she argues, often reflect more general cultural beliefs, attitudes, and understandings. For example, American doctors frequently feel heroic measures are called for in cases where British doctors may feel that the most appropriate line of action is to let things "run their course."[12]

But, of course, it cannot be denied that the widespread acceptance of the appropriateness of the medical model as the major schema for interpreting infertility must necessarily make the experience of infertility in industrial societies radically different from that of nonindustrial societies. There is a fundamental difference between the medical model of illness and its more traditional models: the former sharply distinguishes between the technical and the interpretive aspects of health problems, while the latter do not. The medical model is self-consciously secular. Medical practitioners explain illness in both physical and psychological terms, but they see questions of ultimate significance as largely irrelevant to understanding health problems and to practicing healing.[13]

In Chapter 2, I argue that infertility, like other aspects of reproduction,[14] is in the process of becoming *medicalized;* that is, the medical model is becoming the dominant cognitive framework in terms of which sufferers interpret their experience. A major purpose of this book is to demonstrate the ways in which the medicalization of infertility has contributed to transforming the experience of infertility. It is not my purpose here to argue that the medical approach to infertility is wrong; rather, I assert that it is one approach among many and that its acceptance has had a dramatic impact on the nature of the infertility experience.

SOCIAL STRUCTURE AND THE
EXPERIENCE OF INFERTILITY

My discussion of the cultural variability of practices and beliefs associated with infertility may have given the impression that there is no rhyme or reason to this variability. If we look at a culture's beliefs and practices regarding infertility in its social and cultural contexts, however, we see that this is not the case.

Among the best documented practices and beliefs concerning infertility are those of the Ndembu of Zambia, described by anthropologist Victor Turner in a series of well-known works. The Ndembu have four separate rituals that deal with infertility. A woman who has been unable to conceive or to bring a pregnancy to term consults a diviner, who, after conducting a seance attended by the woman's kin and possibly her neighbors, reveals the cause of the problem and recommends which of the four available ritual solutions should be used to alleviate it. The afflicted woman is almost always diagnosed as having been "caught" by the shade of a maternal ancestor; often her mother or maternal grandmother, offended by the woman's actions, has come out of her grave to "sit" in the woman's body. The purpose of the ritual, which involves not only the wife but usually also her husband and maternal and paternal relatives, is to propitiate the shade who has been obstructing the woman's fertility. Once a woman has completed the ritual, the shade who had obstructed her fertility now protects it; then the woman, her husband, and other close male relatives are eligible to become adepts in the ritual cult and may administer the ritual to others.[15]

Why are the Ndembu inclined to attribute infertility to an offense against one's own maternal ancestors? If we accept Turner's analysis of the situation, the answer has little to do with medicine and much to do with social structure. Ndembu society is characterized by matrilineal descent ideology and virilocal residence. In plain English, a woman owes her primary allegiance to her own maternal kin, but when she is married, she goes to live with her husband and his kin; thus, a source of tension is built into Ndembu society. A woman's loyalties are often divided between her own kin to whom she theoretically owes her primary allegiance and her husband's kin with whom she lives. Not surprisingly, her own maternal kin often feel that they are not getting the attention due them.

There is, if you will, a fault line running through Ndembu social life. When a woman fails to conceive and people try to understand why, their attention is naturally drawn to this major source of tension within the society. Infertility is seized upon by the Ndembu as an occasion for working through structural tensions that, on the face of it, have nothing to do with infertility. Thus, to understand the Ndembu's experience of infertility, one must understand the nature of the structural crises built into Ndembu society.

Likewise, the experience of infertility in contemporary American society is shaped by our own set of structural tension points. Three of those tension points are especially important to understand the contemporary experience of infertility: intimate relations within marriage, the power of the medical profession and public confidence in it, and the quest for an enduring system of meaning that stands over and above the individual.

First, we are living in a time when role expectations for men and women are changing, not fast enough for some, too fast for others. What Carl Degler calls "the doctrine of the two spheres"—that is, the ideology stating that the appropriate roles for husbands to play within the family are those of "provider," "protector," and "disciplinarian" while the appropriate roles for wives are those of "caretaker," "household manager," and "emotional specialist"—is losing much of its authority.[16] Wives and husbands often find that the scripts for which they have been socialized are neither the scripts they desire to play nor those their spouses expect them to play. At an interpersonal level, this means that husbands and wives are often uncertain of what to expect of each other.

Americans today demand much of the family as a social institution. We ask it to be a "haven in a heartless world," to provide us with the intimacy missing in so many of our other social relationships.[17] One must question whether any social institution, even under the best of circumstances, could live up to such high expectations. One major strain on contemporary marriage may stem from the fact that we simply desire too much from it. But marital relationships are further strained by the fact that the different socialization experiences of women and men in American society have led to differences in wives' and husbands' needs for communication and intimacy.[18] Different styles of intimacy for women and men in turn give rise to what Lilian Rubin calls the "approach-avoidance script" of American marriages: wives press for greater intimacy and emotional support through talk while husbands wonder what there is to say.[19]

Infertility is a health problem that, because it affects both members of the marital couple, requires much communication and mutual decision making. Thus, wives' and husbands' experiences of infertility are likely to reflect and, perhaps, exacerbate the tensions already present in American marriages.[20]

A second structural tension point in American society concerns our reluctant dependence on medical institutions. During the course of the twentieth century, the medical profession has attained a monopoly over our understanding of the nature of health and illness as well as control over how people defined as sick are treated. In *The Social Transformation of American Medicine*, Paul Starr traces the process by which American medicine became the profession par excellence in American society. And in *The Medicalization of Deviance*, sociologists Peter Conrad and Joseph Schneider show how more and more aspects of our lives are becoming defined as medical problems with medical solutions. Yet, the pedestal upon which American medicine sits has been described as clay, and there are signs that medicine's privileged place in our lives and our minds may be crumbling.[21]

A number of scathing critiques have been launched against contemporary medical institutions.[22] Consumers, corporations, and health insurance providers complain about high costs and an inefficient organizational structure.[23] Patients express dissatisfaction with their doctors and the ways in which their doctors treat them.[24] Perhaps the high rates of noncompliance with doctors' orders reflect this dissatisfaction.[25] But, for all our griping, most of us still embrace, in whole or in part, the medical profession's understanding of health and illness. And reluctantly or not, we still rely on our doctors when we are sick. For their part, doctors feel beleaguered—expressing concern over high rates of patient noncompliance and the high cost of malpractice insurance and in general charging that the public expects too much from them.

Americans define infertility as a medical problem, and infertile couples most often turn to the medical profession for a solution. Thus, not unexpectedly the experiences of infertile couples are shaped to a large degree by the tensions characterizing contemporary medicine.[26]

A third structural tension point in contemporary American society concerns questions of ultimate significance—questions about how we are to make sense of our lives, how we are to choose what goals to strive for. Such questions of meaning and purpose have traditionally been viewed as the sphere of religion. Answers to questions concerning ultimate significance usually refer to the idea of God or—more generally—to the realm of the sacred. In the best-selling *Habits of the Heart*, sociologist Robert Bellah and his associates argue that Americans lack a sense of moral purpose beyond the level of individual experience and interpersonal relationships.[27]

In *The Sacred Canopy*, another sociologist, Peter Berger, posits that in contemporary society industrialism, bureaucracy, and competitive visions of reality have transformed the attempt to construct sacred meaning systems into a precarious undertaking.[28] The rise of industrialism has led many to question the validity of any idea that cannot be subjected to empirical testing. The rise of bureaucratic capitalism has given plausibility to the notion that all enterprises can be judged by reference to such economic ideas as efficiency and costs and benefits. The existence of a multitude of subcultures, each with its own method of making sense of the world, has prompted many to wonder whether any one way can be right.

Still, few social scientists accept the notion that the decline of sacred meaning systems is inevitable in industrial societies. People seemingly need to make sense out of their lives. As their realities are threatened by experience, they begin the process of constructing new realities. Thus at the same time that the industrialism, bureaucracy, and pluralism of contemporary society are threatening the mainline churches, the traditional institutional bases of meaning in American society, people are turning to conservative religion, cults, alternative healing groups, and the New Age movement in attempts to find moral guidelines in a confusing time.

Infertility is experienced by infertile couples as personal and family tragedy, a threat to long-standing assumptions about the meaning and direction of their lives. Therefore, the experience of infertility will be significantly affected by the sense of moral uncertainty pervading contemporary American society.[29]

At the same time, then, that this book describes the experience of infertile couples, it likewise discusses gender relations, people's reactions to their encounters with medical treatment, and attempts of ordinary, middle-class Americans to make sense out of their lives. In the course of describing the experiences of infertile couples and highlighting the reasons they respond to their situations as they do, I also aim to provide the reader with a window on important tensions that exist within American social institutions.

As I pursue this theoretical agenda, I hope to accomplish some practical aims as well. Infertile readers stand to benefit greatly from realizing that much of their experience is typical and normal, given the social-structural context of infertility in contemporary America. Additional insight into the experience of infertility may help doctors, counselors, friends, and relatives be more responsive to the needs of infertile couples. Finally, a better understanding of the social context of the experience of infertility should help shed light on current policy debates surrounding such issues as surrogate motherhood, reproductive technology, and adoption.

METHODS

My data for this book come from several sources. I depend primarily on a study in which two colleagues and I interviewed twenty-two married, infertile couples in western New York State (data collection is described below). In my interpretations of the interview material, I have relied on several other sources of information as well. Some interpretations depend on insights derived from the quantitative analysis of health history questionnaires administered to 449 couples at an infertility clinic in central New York State.[30] I have also undertaken an extensive review of literature in the fields of sociology, psychology, anthropology, history, social policy, social work, medicine, and nursing that touches on the experience of infertile couples. Finally, I am a member of an infertile couple, and much of what I write is illuminated by our own experiences and by those recounted to us informally by infertile friends and acquaintances.

Decisions about the Research Design

The most important research design decisions—answers to fundamental questions about who one wishes to study and what it is about them one would like to learn—must, of course, be made long before one ventures into the field. In the case of my research, I had two particularly important decisions to make: first, whether to use a questionnaire or structured interview format as opposed to a relatively unstructured format; and, second whether to focus on infertile individuals or on infertile *couples*.[31]

The literature on the social-psychological impact of infertility is by now growing rapidly.[32] Most studies are, however, based on the quantitative analysis of responses to structured questions. In quantitative analysis, researchers conceptualize reality as an array of set characteristics called "variables." The variables a researcher chooses to study are determined by what the researcher has learned to think of as relevant to the research problem. To tap these areas of presumed reality, social science researchers write precise, carefully worded questions with a strictly limited range of acceptable answers. The data that result from such a procedure are reliable, but they are often quite far removed from the actual experience of the supposed subjects of the research. Quantitative studies can show us that one variable is statistically related to another, but they can seldom

17

provide much insight into how people go about making sense of their lives.

It is a basic tenet of the symbolic interactionist approach in sociology that the most important goal of social science is to understand how people come to define and interpret their experience. The methodological approach generally regarded as best suited to generating data about how people make sense of social reality is known as "grounded theory."[33] A researcher using grounded theory neither brings to the data a set of preconceived categories to be imposed upon them nor necessarily has a clear hypothesis about how these categories may relate to one another. Rather, grounded theory supplies a set of inductive techniques for drawing categories *out* of data.

I decided to gather my data by means of relatively unstructured interviews that I planned to analyze qualitatively rather than quantitatively. I opted for this approach because I wanted to capture the texture of the experienced realities of infertile couples, and I thought I would be better able to do this if I allowed them to speak about their own concerns in their own words. I did not want them to have to squeeze their experience into conceptual boxes I had made for them; I wanted to let them speak for themselves.

Other researchers have employed the qualitative analysis of unstructured interviews as a means of gaining insight into the experience of infertility, but most of these researchers have either exclusively or primarily focused on women.[34] I was interested in studying both members of infertile couples because I knew that infertility has a powerful impact on the couple as a unit. Thus, it was relatively easy to decide that I needed to interview both partners in an infertile couple, regardless of who was diagnosed as reproductively impaired. Next I considered whether to interview the couple together or whether to interview each partner separately.

In *The Future of Marriage*, Jessie Bernard used the term "'his' and 'her' marriages" to drive home her point that husbands' and wives' experiences of the same marriage are often quite different. The contention that husbands and wives are often less than perfectly aware of each other's perceptions of the dynamics of family life is by now well documented by research in the sociology of the family.[35] Although few data have been collected on the question of men's and women's reactions to infertility, what little evidence there is suggests that husbands and wives do react differently.[36] Knowing that wives and husbands were likely to have different reactions and not wanting the responses of one to influence the responses of the other, I elected to interview wives and husbands separately.

Because I did not want wives and husbands to compare notes between their interviews, I opted to work with a team of interviewers who could travel to couples' homes and interview both partners separately but at the same time. I decided to interview couples in their homes, partly for the convenience of the people who agreed to give up their time and privacy to talk to me and partly because I thought people might feel more comfortable talking to a stranger about very private matters if they were able to do so in comfortable surroundings.

Sampling Strategy and Questions of Access

Even in exploratory, qualitative research, the researcher is interested in selecting a sample that is as similar in as many ways as possible to the population about which he or she wishes to generalize. The ideal method for achieving such representativeness is a simple random sample. Obviously this strategy could not be used in a study of this nature. There is, of course, no list of all infertile couples from which to draw a sample, and—even if such a list were available from a clinic or a doctor's office—I did not regard it as ethically acceptable to obtain information of such a private nature about people without their prior consent.

Instead I used a "snowball" sampling technique. I made initial contacts through the local chapter of Resolve, an infertility support organization. I explained my project to the board and asked board members to ask people they knew if they would be willing to be interviewed and to give me the names of those who said "yes." In this way, I located couples to interview without feeling that I was invading their privacy. After I interviewed those first couples, I asked them, in turn, to ask couples they knew about their willingness to be interviewed.

I did not accept more than two referrals from any one respondent, and I encouraged respondents to help locate people not involved in Resolve. Of the twenty-two couples interviewed, twelve reported that at least one member of the couple was active in Resolve.

Using the snowball sampling technique, I interviewed twenty-two couples during the summers of 1985 and 1986. I also made contact with six other couples who had originally agreed to be interviewed but later changed their minds and declined. Early in the process I discovered that when I phoned the couple husbands were more likely than wives to decline to be interviewed, so I made it my practice always to ask for the wife by name. After I spoke to the wives, explaining who I was and reminding them that they had agreed to be interviewed, they often admitted that they had agreed without asking their husbands. "Give me another week to break it to him gently" was a remark I frequently heard.

My most harrowing telephone experience came toward the end of the study as I was talking to a wife, making final arrangements for an interview. Her husband took the phone from her in midsentence and said, "Look, I agreed to this, but if you ask one thing that I find offensive, you're out the door." Needless to say, I approached that interview with some trepidation. As it turned out, the interview went fine, and the suspicious husband turned out to be a thoughtful and insightful respondent.

Couple Characteristics

The couples in my sample were considerably better off than the national average in terms of annual family income and education. The mean estimate of family income given by men was $48,000, by women, $38,000.[37] Of the women, fifteen had completed college as had sixteen of the men; eight women and six men had attained advanced degrees; the remainder were high school graduates. All the husbands and thirteen wives were engaged in full-time employment outside the home at the time of the interview. Eighteen husbands and ten wives worked in professional or managerial positions. All couples were white.

It is clear that this sample is not representative of the U.S. infertile population as a whole. Although the couples in my sample are white and above average in terms of income and education, reproductive impairments are actually more common among blacks and those with lower incomes.[38] Presumably these couples have much greater access to medical and other resources for coping with infertility and greater exposure to infertility treatment than the infertile population at large. Furthermore, many of my respondents are active in Resolve; they are surely different in some significant ways from those who do not join self-help groups. Participation in Resolve may have led them to define and interpret their infertility quite differently from non-Resolve members. Even those who are not Resolve members are seekers of treatment, likely to be significantly different from infertile couples who have not sought treatment.

The nonrepresentativeness of my sample is by and large an artifact of my sampling strategy. I know of no other published studies of infertile couples based on intensive interviews with both partners of marital couples that do not share the same sampling biases, but comparisons between my findings and those reported by researchers who have conducted intensive interviews among clinic-based samples of women and by researchers who tried to include black and lower SES women in their samples lead me to believe that many of my findings may be more generalizable than one might initially suspect.[39] Like my study, these other interview-based studies focus virtually exclusively on treatment-seekers. The problem of how feasibly to gain access to those who have not sought treatment is difficult to solve. It would be unwise to assume that any generalizations I make in this book necessarily apply to those who have not sought treatment.

According to wives' estimates, the average duration of infertility at the time of the interview was 6.7 years; according to husbands' estimates, it was 5.2 years.[40] My sample included couples with a wide range of medical, reproductive, and family growth histories. Infertility was due to a female reproductive impairment in nine cases, to a male reproductive impairment in four, and to a combination of male and female reproductive impairments in six. In the remaining three cases, the source of the couple's infertility had not been identified. Three of the twenty-two couples had biological children prior to their involvement with infertility; therefore, they are classified as cases of secondary infertility.

Of nineteen couples who were involuntarily childless at the start of their infertility treatment, eleven couples had adopted children by the time of the interview. One wife had had a successful pregnancy, and four wives (including two who had already adopted at least one child) were aware of being pregnant at the time of the interview. By the time of the interview fourteen couples had achieved some measure of success in their quests for children.

There are at least two possible reasons for the high proportion of adoptive parents in my sample. First, the longer couples have been struggling with infertility, the more likely they are to be known to others. The snowball sampling technique would, therefore, be more likely to identify couples who had adopted children. In fact, neighbors and acquaintances do not know many couples are infertile until they have adopted a child. Second, once contacted, "successful" couples may have been more likely to agree to be interviewed. To be infertile is to occupy a stigmatized social status,[41] and couples who perceived themselves as "failures" in the infertility process may have been less willing to be interviewed.

Conduct of the Interview

All interviews were taped. Interviewers advised respondents that their voices were being taped and assured them that the contents of the interview would be kept confidential.

Although the process by which I obtained permission to interview a couple was not always straightforward and hassle-free, once the interviewing team arrived at a couple's house, it was usually quite easy to establish rapport. As we will see, many wives were accustomed to spending considerable time talking about infertility; many said that talking to us was not terribly unlike talking with an infertile friend. Their husbands were less used to talking about infertility but seemed, for the most part, to relax soon after the interview began. The other interviewers and I are convinced that all our respondents, wives and husbands, spoke frankly with us.

Surprisingly enough, taping the interviews seemed to make it easier to establish rapport, especially with the husbands. Because we did not want to lug around heavy and obtrusive equipment, we used miniaturized recording equipment. In general, husbands were so fascinated by our equipment that our little microcassette recorders served as icebreakers as well as recording devices.

Interviews were of the type known in sociology as the "focused interview." Interviewers, though guided by a list of questions to be asked, were free to vary the order and the wording of the questions, based on their judgments about how the interview was progressing. The interview guide can be found in the Appendix. Interviews lasted an average of an hour and a quarter. Subjects included the decision to bear children, treatment history, reactions to treatment, decisions regarding adoption and reproductive technologies, couple reaction to infertility, changes in life-style and social relationships, effects of infertility and infertility decision making on career, and effects of infertility on values, attitudes, and world view. Interviewers were careful to be sensitive and responsive to respondents' comments rather than judgmental. Our obvious familiarity with common reactions to infertility and our obvious recognition and comprehension of such medical terms as laparoscopy and hysterosalpingogram helped, I think, to convince our respondents that we understood what they were going through and that it was alright to level with us.

Although most couples interviewed had children in the home by the time of the interview, they generally (excluding, of course, the three cases of secondary infertility) exhibited a strong tendency to discuss their "pre-child" days at great length. Thus, to the extent that respondents discussed what they *had* experienced rather than what they were currently experiencing, these data suffer from some drawbacks that characterize all retrospective data. Moreover, individuals who survey the past from the vantage point of present success may develop strikingly different accounts from those who view it from the perspective of continued failure. Like all data collected by interview techniques, the data reported upon here must be understood as couples' interpretative *accounts* of their attitudes and behaviors rather than as objective records of those attitudes and behaviors.

Occasionally during the course of the interviews respondents would ask the interviewers what they thought about a particular topic that had been raised. When this happened, the interviewers told the respondents that they did not want to say anything that might influence the respondents' discussions during the course of the interview but that they would be happy to answer any questions after the interview. When the interview was over, all respondents, whether they had expressed interest or not, were given an opportunity to ask the interviewers anything they wished. Usually they asked us how we became interested in infertility, what we planned to do with the results, and such personal questions as whether we were married, had children, and so on. We answered all such questions honestly. Both the other infertile interviewer and I told respondents at this point in the interview that we were infertile and discussed our personal experiences with infertility.

At this point in the interview, one wife asked me if I would contact her later to tell her what her husband had said. I replied that to do so would violate my promise of confidentiality to him and that, if she wanted to know what he had said, she would have to ask him directly.

A few times during the course of the interviews people made statements that led the interviewers to think that they were misinformed, either about the basis of a diagnosis, the proper treatment for certain conditions, opportunities for adoption, or some other issue concerning the process of infertility decision making. These occasions presented me with a moral quandary. On the one hand, I did not feel it was my place as a researcher to tell people who were confiding in a stranger that I felt their course of action was inappropriate. On the other hand, I did not feel that it was ethical to say nothing when I suspected a couple might harm themselves by acting on what I thought was misinformation. Our strategy on these few occasions was to wait until the end of the interview to raise the subject. When we did raise the subject, we tried to do so in such a way that did not imply that we were medical experts. Rather than say, "I think you're making a mistake about x," we tried to say something more on the order of, "You might want to ask your doctor about x," or "I know a good article about x," or "I have a friend who went through x whom you might want to talk to."

Throughout the interviewing process I tried to keep in mind that research at its best is reciprocal. I feel that my respondents helped me by consenting to open up their lives for me; then it was my duty, not only not to harm them, but also to see that they gained from the experience. I hope that when they see the book I have written they will feel I have repaid some of the debt I owe them.

OUTLINE OF THE BOOK

I have tried to write this book in a way that reflects the inductive style in which I carried out the research. I begin each chapter with description, trying to sketch out the patterns I discern among the twenty-two couples. As patterns emerge I venture into explanation, trying to account for the configurations I have discovered.

Chapter 2 presents an account of the medicalization of infertility as well as a description of the contemporary medical setting that provides the context for couples' experiences of infertility. In Chapter 3, I turn my attention to the couples themselves for the first time and focus on their feelings about their bodies and themselves, paying special attention to differences between husbands and wives. In Chapter 4, I describe infertile couples' encounters with medical professionals and their experiences of the treatment regimen. Chapter 5 examines the effects of infertility on the marital relationship, while Chapter 6 looks at infertility's effects on social relationships in general. In Chapter 7, I describe couples' attempts to place their experience of infertility within a broader framework of meaning.

Finally, in Chapter 8, I deal systematically with the issues I raised earlier in this chapter about the relationship between infertility and its social context. How do contemporary social institutions help shape the contemporary experience of infertility? Conversely, what can examining the experience of infertility tell us about social strains within American society? I conclude with a brief discussion of the practical implications of my analysis for delivering health care to infertile couples and forming social policy.

TWO

INFERTILITY AS A
MEDICAL CONDITION
Social and Historical Contexts

I t is impossible to say exactly how many American couples are like Liz and Matt and the other couples I interviewed, but it seems clear that they have plenty of company. By defining infertility as failure to conceive after twelve months of unprotected intercourse, demographer William Mosher estimates on the basis of data collected as part of the National Survey of Family Growth that 2.4 million married couples were infertile in 1982.[1] This figure represents 8.5 percent of all married couples at that time; however, it represents 13.9 percent of all married couples who have not chosen to undergo surgical intervention (e.g., a vasectomy or tubal ligation) to prevent conception. Mosher's estimate of 2.4 million infertile couples is almost certainly too low because he does not account for the existence of hidden infertility: that is, some women, especially those in lower age brackets, have never had intercourse unprotected by contraceptive devices and have therefore never tested their fertility.

If hidden infertility were taken into account, the proportion of infertile couples might come closer to or even exceed the 15 percent estimated by Barbara Eck Menning, founder of Resolve.[2] Even this figure does not include couples who may have at some time in the past had difficulty conceiving. When one considers that 37.5 percent of all childless women fail to conceive within twelve months of unprotected intercourse and that 16 percent of *all planned pregnancies* occur after a period of twelve months or longer of unprotected intercourse, then the proportion of American couples who have experienced infertility at some point in their lives may be very large indeed.[3]

Not all infertile couples are childless. Medical practitioners generally differentiate between "primary infertility," or involuntary childlessness, and "secondary infertility," or infertility experienced by couples who already have at least one biological child. Hirsch and Mosher estimate that primary infertility accounts for only 30 percent of infertility among American couples.[4] In other words, 70 percent of American infertile couples already have at least one biological child in the home.

MEDICAL TREATMENT OF INFERTILITY

Not all infertile couples look for medical solutions to their problem. In fact, the majority of U.S. infertile couples do not seek treatment. Of the women identified as infertile in 1982 by the National Survey of Family Growth, 43.7 percent reported that they had been to a physician or a clinic to seek treatment. Women with primary infertility are approximately twice as likely as those with secondary infertility to seek treatment. Although reproductive impairments are actually more common among blacks and those with lower incomes, whites and those with higher incomes are most likely to seek treatment.[5]

The fact that infertility is more common among the disadvantaged while access to treatment is greater among the relatively well-off should not surprise us; it reflects a basic well-documented fact about health and health care in American society: those with higher levels of educational and economic attainment enjoy both better health and better access to health care.[6]

All the couples I interviewed have either been treated for infertility in the past or are currently being treated. The experience of treatment, an important part of the experience of infertility, helps give that experience its distinctive character. Because the couples I spoke with often talked about their treatment regimens, it will help the reader to be at least somewhat familiar with the diagnostic tests and medical treatments that these couples have undergone.

In approximately 80 to 90 percent of couples who present themselves for medical treatment it is possible to discover a clear medical reason (or reasons) for a couple's infertility.[7] Although the general public tends to see infertility as the woman's problem,[8] the husband or the wife or both may have the reproductive impairment. Most studies of people attending infertility clinics have reported that a male factor is involved in 20 to 40 percent of those cases where a cause for the failure to conceive can be identified. It is therefore necessary to consider both partners during the course of medical investigations of infertility.

Investigations of female reproductive impairments may be complicated and usually take a number of months to complete. The infertility workup typically starts with a physical examination and a detailed medical history. One of the first diagnostic procedures recommended to women being treated for infertility is charting basal body temperature (BBT). In the BBT regimen, the woman takes her temperature upon awakening each morning and marks it on a chart. If her basal body temperature rises at about the middle of the menstrual cycle, then she is probably ovulating. BBT charts give the physician a crude indication of ovulatory problems and also make sure that the infertile couple is engaging in intercourse during that part of the cycle when conception is most likely.

Another test of ovulation, often included in the initial infertility workup, is the endometrial biopsy. For that tissue is scraped from the endometrium, the lining of the uterus, and examined for evidence that ovulation has taken place. As an outpatient procedure, the endometrial biopsy is generally performed in the doctor's office.

The hysterosalpingogram, used to locate obstructions in the

Fallopian tubes as well as malformations of the uterus, is also part of the routine infertility workup for a woman. In the hysterosalpingo-gram, dye is injected into the Fallopian tubes. The passage of the dye through the tubes is traced through the use of x-ray techniques. Un-til recently, some physicians used the Rubin test, or tubal insuf-flation, to test the functioning of the Fallopian tubes. Currently, however, the hysterosalpingogram is regarded as the procedure of choice.

The postcoital test involves taking a small sample of mucus from a woman's cervix soon after intercourse. The mucus is examined to see if the male's sperm is capable of surviving in the cervix.

The typical female infertility workup now includes a laparoscopy, in which a fiber-optic instrument (laparoscope) is inserted through a small incision on the woman's abdomen. The laparoscope allows the physician to visually examine the reproductive organs. Because the laparoscopy requires general anesthesia, it is typically performed in the hospital.

Somewhere between 30 and 70 percent of diagnosed female re-productive failures can be traced to problems with ovulation. Ovula-tory problems include amenorrhea (failure to menstruate), oligome-norrhea (scanty or infrequent menstruation), and luteal phase defects (failure of the endometrial lining of the uterus to develop properly after ovulation).[9] Ovulation problems are usually treated with drugs, including clomiphene citrate, human menopausal gonadotro-pin (hMG), and gonadotropin releasing hormone (Gn-RH).

Most remaining diagnosed reproductive problems affecting wo-men involve blockage of the Fallopian tubes. Attempts may be made to repair these blockages surgically; alternatively in vitro fertilization (IVF) may be used to bypass the damaged tubes. In 10 to 30 percent of diagnosed cases, infertility may be related to endometriosis—the presence of endometrial tissue outside the uterus, often in the Fallo-pian tubes or on the ovaries. Endometriosis can be treated surgically or through drug therapy. Usually the drug of choice is danazol, a synthetic derivative of testosterone. Infertility may also be related to uterine malformations, overproduction of the hormone prolactin, infections, and antibodies in the cervical mucus, among other possibilities.

Investigation of male reproductive impairments typically begins with a physical examination, medical history, and semen analysis. In semen analysis, the patient collects a sample of sperm through masturbation. The semen sample is evaluated to determine, among other things, if there is an adequate volume of semen and a sufficient concentration of sperm and if the spermatozoa are sufficiently active (or motile) and normal in structure (or morphology). If the results of the semen analysis are normal, no further tests are performed. If semen analysis reveals abnormalities, an evaluation of hormone levels will typically be undertaken. Other tests that may sometimes be conducted include a testicular biopsy and x-ray examination of the sperm transport ducts.

Male reproductive impairments are sometimes treated with hormone therapy, but its usefulness is not yet clear. For certain specific male reproductive problems, surgery may be appropriate. The most common surgical procedure performed on men is varicocele repair, or varicocelectomy. Varicoceles, dilute varicose veins in the testes, are fairly common, but they are found more frequently in men with reproductive impairments than in those without fertility problems. Varicocelectomy involves tying off the varicose vein.

One common treatment for male fertility problems is artificial insemination. Artificial insemination by husband (AIH) is sometimes used in cases where a man produces some viable sperm. It is often used in conjunction with techniques such as sperm washing or the swim-up technique that separate the most viable from the least viable sperm. Artificial insemination by donor (AID) is not a treatment for male infertility but rather a means of bypassing a partner whose reproductive impairments resist correction. In recent years, some clinicians have begun recommending IVF as a treatment for male reproductive impairments.

In approximately 10 to 20 percent of infertile couples, it may not be possible to locate a biomedical cause for the problem. This so-called "normal infertility" is referred to technically as idiopathic infertility. Many couples with idiopathic infertility are currently being referred to IVF programs.

Most studies have found that couples treated for infertility have about a 50 percent chance of achieving a pregnancy.[10] Pregnancy rates for couples whose principle diagnosis is ovulatory problems are much higher than those for other couples,[11] while couples whose principle diagnosis is tubal problems are much less likely to achieve pregnancy. A 50 percent success rate seems quite impressive at first glance, and it certainly gives infertile couples reason to believe that it is worthwhile to pursue treatment. It is important, however, to keep in mind that not all pregnancies experienced by couples undergoing treatment for infertility are in fact treatment-related. A study conducted by physician John A. Collins and his associates found that, while 41 percent of couples treated for infertility subsequently conceived, so did 35 percent of those who had not received treatment.[12] It is therefore not clear that all—or even most—pregnancies achieved by infertile couples pursuing treatment can be definitively linked to the medical treatment process itself.

Infertile women who do become pregnant are more likely to experience pregnancy losses than are other women. For the infertile, the experience of pregnancy is more likely to be surrounded by anxiety and to end in grief.[13]

THE CONCEPT OF MEDICALIZATION

The years since the advent of the first test tube baby in 1978 have seen a dramatic increase in the media's attention to infertility.[14] The media's increased coverage has given many people the impression that the incidence of infertility has been rising dramatically. In fact, this is not the case. According to William Mosher, the incidence of infertility actually declined from 3.0 million in 1965 to 2.4 million in 1982. The number of *childless* infertile couples, however, doubled from 0.5 million to 1.0 million during the same time period.[15] Because female fertility declines with increasing age, the current trend in American society toward delayed childbearing among the middle class means that now a larger percentage of middle-class infertile couples are childless when they discover their infertility. At a time when women started their childbearing careers earlier than they do today, a larger percentage of those who found difficulty conceiving already had children in the home. To summarize the current trend using medical language, although the overall incidence of infertility is not increasing, the proportion of cases of primary infertility, as opposed to secondary infertility, is increasing. Because the tendency to delay childbearing is most pronounced among those with greater educational and occupational attainment,[16] the trend toward an increasing proportion of cases of primary infertility is occurring primarily among the white middle class. Among blacks and those with lower incomes, secondary infertility is more common.[17]

Although the number of infertile couples has not necessarily risen drastically in recent years, the proportion of couples, who—like Liz and Matt and the other people I spoke with—have decided to seek medical treatment *has* increased dramatically. Office visits for infertility almost tripled between 1968 and 1984, rising from about 600,000 to about 1.6 million over fourteen years. During the same time period, membership in the American Fertility Society, the major organization for physicians interested in or specializing in infertility, showed similar increases, rising from about 3,000 in 1968 to almost 10,000 in 1984.[18]

Liz and Matt are typical of many American couples: the female partner initiated the infertility investigation, and she was the subject of the focus of most treatment attempts. While office visits for infertility have increased substantially in recent years among women, men's visits have remained at virtually the same level as before.[19]

One way to describe this trend toward increased treatment rates among infertile couples and increased professional interest in infertility is to say that infertility is in the process of becoming increasingly *medicalized*. Sociologists use the term "medicalization" to describe the process by which certain behaviors come to be understood as questions of health and illness, subject to the authority of medical institutions.[20] For example, the medicalization of alcoholism has meant that it has become defined as an addictive disorder (rather than as a moral failing). Given this definition, residential treatment centers, for example, are becoming seen as the appropriate place to deal with the behavior of alcoholics. Social critic Ivan Illich has used the term "the medicalization of life" to characterize the way in which more and more aspects of social life have come under the influence of medical authority during the twentieth century. Rising treatment rates for infertility seem to indicate that increasing numbers of both sufferers and medical professionals are defining infertility as a primarily medical problem.

The trend toward medicalization in the twentieth century developed as part of a larger trend toward increasing prestige for science and technology. In the early twentieth century, one idea emerged as prevalent in American society: all varieties of human endeavor could be improved upon if they were rationalized and reorganized according to the presumably scientific principles that guided industrial production. Among the fields that certain people attempted to remake in the name of science were social work, education, corrections, and housework.[21] The attempt to organize all manner of enterprise according to the presumed dictates of science and technology implicitly challenged the validity of all approaches to human problems other than the scientific and the technological.

As infertility becomes medicalized, medical institutions and medical world views supply a major context shaping infertile couples' experiences. According to sociologists Peter Conrad and Joseph Schneider, medicalization takes place at three levels: the conceptual, the institutional, and the level of doctor-patient interaction.[22] Defining infertility as a medical problem means that infertility is described in medical language, that it is treated in medical institutions, and that sufferers are regarded as patients. In the following paragraphs, I discuss aspects of the medical approach to reality that seem especially likely to have an impact on couples' experiences of infertility.

To say that a condition or problem has become medicalized is to say, first, that a medical vocabulary becomes employed in describing the condition or problem. A medicalized problem or condition is conceptualized according to the medical model, a secular model that sees the source of disease as primarily organic in nature and excludes nonempirical speculation from consideration. The medical model is based on a technology-inspired image of the human body. The body is seen as analogous to a machine made up of interdependent parts, any one of which can malfunction. Causes of disease other than organic causes existing within the individual are typically considered irrelevant. The focus of the medical model is not so much on the person considered as a whole as on the diseased organ. Treatment seeks to eliminate or manage the diseased condition.[23]

When a problem or condition becomes medicalized, sufferers become subject to cultural beliefs about the nature of illness and the proper role for the sick. In the United States, these include the belief that the sufferer should do everything in his or her power to get better.[24] Another belief that seems to be spreading in contemporary Western societies is the idea that the individual is ultimately responsible for his or her own condition.[25] Sufferers are also affected by widespread respect for achievement and the concomitant stigmatization of illness.[26]

I now turn to the institutional level of medicalization: a medicalized condition or problem becomes the province of autonomous medical specialists, who have the exclusive right and obligation to diagnose and treat it. The problem or condition simultaneously becomes subject to the institutional constraints of professional medicine. American medicine, organized as a profit-making enterprise, is financed to a large extent through the mechanism of health insurance. Health problems are typically treated in hospitals, clinics, doctors' offices, and other facilities specifically dedicated to medical purposes. The focus of medical attention is more often on the cure of the disease rather than its prevention and on acute rather than chronic illness.[27]

Medicalization also takes place at the level of doctor-patient interaction. When a problem or condition becomes medicalized, the sufferer (or, at least, the sufferer who seeks treatment) becomes a patient, subject to the conditions of doctor-patient interaction, including a passive role for the patient and dominance over face-to-face interaction by the physician.[28]

Because the medicalization of infertility is currently affecting women more than men and because infertile women are typically treated by gynecologists, it's worth noting several aspects of gynecological practice that may be expected to have an influence on the experience of infertility. A number of writers have noted the tendency of gynecologists to view women's behavior as largely determined by their reproductive organs; therefore, they see women as more passive and less intellectually oriented than men. Historians of obstetrics have noted the development among obstetricians of the idea that birth is a pathological process requiring constant monitoring and frequent intervention. Sociologist Diane Scully has called attention to the interventionist orientation of gynecology, noting that the gynecological residents she studied saw learning to do surgery as the most important part of their training.[29]

THE MEDICALIZATION OF INFERTILITY

One sphere of life that has become increasingly medicalized during the course of the twentieth century is reproduction, especially women's reproductive lives.[30] First, in the early twentieth century, midwives lost out to doctors as "social birth" was replaced by medical birth and as home birth was replaced by hospital birth. Since that time, pregnancy, contraception, abortion, and menopause have all become defined as medical questions, subject to medical understanding and physicians' control. One crude indication of the extent to which reproduction has been medicalized is the fact that, as of 1981, 61.9 percent of all visits to gynecologists were for reasons not related to illness.[31]

We must not assume that the medicalization of reproduction has been simply rammed down women's throats by a medical profession anxious to expand its sphere of influence. Sociologist Catherine

Kohler Riessman has suggested that the medicalization of reproduction has occurred when doctors' interests to maximize their professional power has converged with women's perceptions of their own medical needs, especially among relatively affluent white women.[32] With regard to the medicalization of birth, for example, women were willing to leave their homes for the hospital because "twilight sleep" offered them some possible relief from the pain of childbirth. According to Riessman, the medicalization of reproduction has proceeded when the medical profession's interests to expand its jurisdiction has fit with the desire of women to free their bodies from control by biological processes. But the medicalization of reproduction, according to Riessman, is ironic: at the same time that it has promised women more control over their bodies, it has strengthened the control of the biomedical interpretation of their experience. In recent years, the profession of obstetrics and gynecology has seen itself criticized by women who challenge its right to dominate the interpretation and management of reproductive health.[33]

Historical sociologist Adele Clarke argues that reproduction has been not simply *medicalized* but *industrialized* as well.[34] By saying that reproduction has become industrialized, Clarke intends to convey its subjection to rational control via the same techniques brought to bear in factory production. Childbirth, for example has become an enterprise of mass production, supervised by trained specialists, dependent upon expensive and sophisticated equipment, and managed according to principles of rational efficiency. Contraception, too, has become a planned, rational, affair that relies on mass-produced products and the services of experts. Some aspects of reproduction have become industrialized faster than others. According to Clarke, industrialization has proceeded more rapidly in those reproductive processes for which a product can be mass-produced or services can be feasibly delivered on a mass scale, and those for which a large market is perceived.

I interpret the recent increases in both the provision and the utilization of infertility services as evidence that the medical industrialization of infertility has now begun in earnest. In the paragraphs that follow, I attempt to use the theoretical insights developed by Riessman and Clarke to shed some light on why the medical industrialization of infertility is occurring now.

Obviously medical services cannot undergo expansion unless there is a preexisting demand for those services or unless demand is developed. In the case of infertility, it appears that there has been a longstanding demand for medical services. Historian Judith Schneid Lewis reports that helping women become pregnant was considered by patients to be a major function of the aristocratic *accoucheurs*, forerunners of modern-day obstetricians, who served the British aristocracy in the late eighteenth and early nineteenth centuries.[35] In the mid-nineteenth century, J. Marion Sims, often regarded as the father of modern gynecology, was reportedly constantly "being besieged by unhappy women whose one dominant desire was to have offspring, even at the cost of major operations and all kinds of personal discomfort."[36]

In the 1930s infertile women wrote to the Children's Bureau in Washington requesting advice about how to get medical assistance, and, in the 1940s and 1950s women wrote to the reproductive endocrinologist John Rock volunteering to serve as guinea pigs for any experimental therapy that might offer some hope. In 1956, *Science Digest* reported that physicians were complaining because infertile women, desperate to have a baby, were "shopping" from doctor to doctor.[37]

Nineteenth-century accoucheurs and gynecologists apparently saw caring for infertile patients as a legitimate part of their responsibilities, but they did not have much to offer. In the 1830s the repertoire of cures offered to Lady Augusta Fox by her accoucheur included "change of air," sea bathing, sexual abstinence, and rest.[38] From the mid-nineteenth century through the early twentieth century, most cases of female infertility were attributed to displacements of the uterus, which were treated surgically in some cases and manipulated without surgery in others.[39] Some cases of infertility were attributed to cervical stenosis, an abnormal narrowing of the cervical canal, and were treated sometimes with surgery and sometimes with more conservative means.

Around the middle of the nineteenth century, Sims, one of the first physicians who realized that the microscope could be more than just a plaything, demonstrated that men as well as women could have reproductive impairments when he discovered dead spermatozoa in a sample of mucus taken from a woman's cervix immediately after intercourse.[40] Sims experimented with artificial insemination, based on this discovery, but he had little success with it because he and his contemporaries did not know at which point in the menstrual cycle conception is possible. Describing infertility, one physician wrote in 1894, "in no condition is the prognosis more uncertain."[41] The early twentieth century saw some major advances in the diagnosis of female infertility, including the development of x-ray techniques and the invention of the Rubin test for tubal patency. Although tubal problems could now be accurately diagnosed, in most cases it was still not possible to treat them successfully.

The fact that gynecologists lacked successful therapies for infertility does not in and of itself explain why the medical profession did not try to colonize this area of treatment more aggressively. After all, physicians were trying to drive midwives out of the birth process long before it was possible to supply any evidence that they could do a better job than those they wished to supplant.[42] Why, then, was there not a greater expansion of infertility services in the nineteenth and early twentieth centuries?

First, it is possible that physicians had more pressing concerns. While infertile women represented a market that comprised 10 to 15 percent of women of reproductive age, pregnant women represented a much larger and still undeveloped market. Second, while labor and delivery services were, in most cases, relatively routine and therefore relatively easy to standardize, the correction of infertility problems, either through surgery or manual manipulation, required the skills of a master. Third, childbirth was typically a successful event for which credit could be claimed, but the same could not be said for infertility. We must remember, too, that before the development of large-scale health insurance schemes in the 1930s the services of specialists were beyond the reach of many.[43] In addition, as one woman complained to the Children's Bureau, those who lived far from cities were unable to obtain the services of specialists.

What, then, did the infertile couples who did not visit gynecologists do about their problem in the nineteenth and early twentieth centuries? Unfortunately, the history of women's and men's reproductive strategies remains to be written. At this time we can only speculate on the basis of some rather piecemeal evidence. Perhaps some women continued to use some of the herbal remedies employed in America and England in the eighteenth century. Perhaps some followed the advice of William Potts Dewees, who noted in 1825 that eating cooked dog meat could make a sterile woman fertile. We have no way of knowing how many infertile women used patent medicines like Lydia Pinkham's Vegetable Compound, which proclaimed at one point in its advertising history that "there's a baby in every bottle." We know that reliance on nonmedical cures for infertility continued well into the twentieth century because we have the testimony of Dr. Allan Roy Dafoe, the physician who delivered the Dionne quintuplets in 1934, that hundreds of sterile women took away "magic pebbles" from the courtyard of the Dionne home in the hope of bearing a child.[44]

In the nineteenth century, people interested in raising children not biologically their own or simply in having children about the house were likely to find it relatively easy to do so. Then, as now, the nuclear family was the dominant family type in American society, but nuclear families were much less insular than they are today. Because men and women often died before the end of their childrearing years,[45] infertile couples were likely to have relatives in need of care. Furthermore, apprenticeship of young children was quite common throughout most of the nineteenth century, and children were frequently hired as workers. Working mothers often placed young children in the homes of both relatives and strangers. Young people moving to new communities typically moved in with a family in the new community.[46] For all these reasons, involuntary childlessness in the nineteenth century was much less likely to mean not having young people around the house than it is today.

Adoption of infants was much less popular as an antidote to childlessness in the first two-thirds of the nineteenth century. Because children were valued more for the labor they could contribute to the household than for their innate "pricelessness," couples preferred to take in older children. As children came to be appreciated more for their sentimental value after 1870, the demand for infants to adopt skyrocketed. By 1910, the demand for adoptable infants exceeded the supply by a ratio of two to one.[47]

Thus, we can surmise that, prior to the industrialization of infertility, many couples used home remedies and domestic strategies in their attempts to deal with infertility. The possibility for the mass delivery of medical infertility services did not become possible until the development of modern conceptions of reproductive endocrinology in the 1920s and 1930s. By 1940, researchers clearly understood the relationship between ovulation and the menstrual cycle; they had isolated the ovarian hormones estrogen and progesterone, determined their functions, and synthesized estrogen in the form of DES.[48]

The development of modern reproductive endocrinology represented a watershed in the history of the medicalization of women's lives. Once they understood the menstrual cycle, physicians wasted little time in attempting to use this knowledge to regulate conception, pregnancy, and menopause. In the mid-1940s, DES began to be used on a fairly widespread basis as a means of preventing miscarriage in the absence of solid evidence that it would be effective for this purpose and in spite of warnings that its use could cause serious problems for DES daughters and sons.[49] The advent of DES made possible the formulation of estrogen replacement therapy as a treatment for menopause. According to sociologist Susan Bell, the development of estrogen replacement therapy and the concomitant conceptualization of menopause as a deficiency disease reinforced cultural stereotypes about the proper role of aging women.[50] The creation of synthetic hormones also made possible the development of the oral contraceptives that became widely used in the 1960s. Although oral contraceptives gave women an unprecedented ability to control conception, they may also pose a long-term threat to women's health. In addition, clear understanding of the menstrual cycle made artificial insemination practical on a mass scale for the first time.

The scientific revolution represented by reproductive endocrinology did not have much practical impact on the treatment of infertility until the mid-1960s. Perusal of the popular literature on infertility in the 1950s reveals that doctors still had few concrete therapies for dealing with infertility. The most effective treatment for infertility in many Ob/Gyn's minds was still to "let nature take her course." This attitude was reinforced by the widespread acceptance in the 1950s of the theories of Dr. Therese Benedek, who wrote that infertility, like most other feminine complaints, was simply emotional rather than medical in its origins.[51]

The early 1960s saw the first clinical trials of clomiphene citrate and hMG, both of which proved highly effective in dealing with ovulatory problems.[52] By the end of the decade, ovulation problems had gone from being a facet of female infertility about which little could be done to being the area in which the highest pregnancy rates were being achieved. We should note that, unlike previously used treatments for infertility, many of which involved surgery, the new hormone therapies were by their very nature cyclical. Unlike surgery, the new hormone therapies could be resorted to month after month if their first use did not result in pregnancy. The late 1960s also saw the development and diffusion of the technique of laparoscopy, which allowed physicians to actually *see* female reproductive impairments.[53] By the end of the 1960s, the technology necessary for the industrialization of infertility was in place.

At this point I should perhaps note that the medicalization of reproduction has probably contributed to the incidence of infertility, against which it is now being directed. DES, intrauterine devices

(IUDs), Caesarean sections, and birth control pills may all be sources of infertility.

The recent expansion of infertility services is sometimes attributed to the development of IVF and other high-tech treatments. It is therefore important to note that the trend toward increased treatment of infertility began well before the first successful attempt at IVF in 1978. It is also worth pointing out that, in terms of technology, too, the development of IVF represents a continuation and acceleration of already developing trends rather than a radical break with the past.

While demand for infertility services already existed prior to the expansion of medical treatment for infertility that began in the late 1960s, certain recent demographic trends may have sharpened that demand. As I have pointed out earlier, the tendency on the part of middle-class American couples to delay childbearing has meant that a larger proportion of middle-class infertile couples is childless than has been the case in the past. Because couples with primary infertility are much more likely to seek treatment than are couples with secondary infertility, we might expect the increase in the proportion of involuntarily childless couples among the middle-class infertile to have resulted in an increased demand for treatment.

Another consequence of the trend toward delayed childbearing is that the window of opportunity for achieving parenthood status has shrunk. With the trend toward delayed childbearing, middle-class women are now more likely to try to condense their childbearing efforts into a shorter period of time than they were previously.[54] Therefore, when these women do discover their infertility, it is likely to occur at an older age when less time remains on the biological clock. Many couples may sense that time is running out: this feeling may also intensify demand.

Although it is clear that American couples have long been disturbed by infertility, the widespread diffusion of birth control technology in the 1960s may have sharpened the edge on couples' dissatisfaction. Many women and men who sought treatment for infertility in the

1970s and 1980s are part of the first generation to come of age in an environment where birth control technology was commonplace and readily available. More important, they are also part of the first generation to come of age believing that the human reproductive process is readily subject to human control.[55] Such people might be more likely to seek treatment than those who doubt their ability to control their reproductive lives.

With regard to this last point, clearly the media's increased attention to the issue of infertility helps popularize the view that infertility is now something controllable. Mass media coverage of infertility emphasizes the promise of such high-tech innovations as IVF and GIFT (gamete inter-Fallopian transfer). "You Don't Have to Be Childless," an article that recently appeared in *Parade Magazine*, concluded: "It's all a question of how much a couple really want a baby; of how much they will pay, how far they will go. Science does have the answers."[56] *Parade*'s acclaim for the prowess of modern, technological medicine strikes me as unjustified. When one considers that only one-half of infertile couples eventually have a child and that less than one-fifth of those undergoing such "miracle cures" eventually give birth, it is clearly an exaggeration to say that anyone who wants a biological baby badly enough can get one.[57]

Also of interest in this regard is work by two anthropologists who conducted a study of the treatment of infertility by traditional healers in Kenya.[58] These anthropologists found that the Kenyan healers had a cure rate of about one-third. The authors suggest that, in some cases of infertility, stress reduction may be more helpful or as helpful as medical intervention. Granted that the 50 percent success rate of Western gynecology is better than the 33 percent claimed by traditional healers, this difference is not so great as to justify the belief that contemporary medical science stands head and shoulders above previous approaches in its ability to treat infertility. Still, the perception that science does have the answers may persuade some couples who might not have pursued treatment several years ago to do so now.

Increased demand for medical services for infertility may also be related to the decreasing availability of nonmedical solutions to the problem of involuntary childlessness, such as adoption. As single parenthood became more acceptable than it had been in the past, the number of healthy white infants available for adoption declined sharply. By 1973, 80 to 90 percent of unwed mothers were keeping their babies. The number of U.S. adoptions decreased from a high of 175,000 in 1970 to 104,000 by 1977, although it seems that the downward trend has since leveled off. [59]

At this point, it is worth mentioning several factors that may have affected the availability of providers of medical services for infertility. Between 1957 and 1976, the total fertility rate in the United States sank from an all-time high of 3,625 to an all-time low of 1,738. [60] There were 4,308,000 births in 1957, but by 1975 this figure had dropped by 27 percent to 3,144,000. [61] This decline has naturally depressed the demand for obstetrical services. At the same time, the number of obstetricians and gynecologists in the United States has risen dramatically. Membership in the American College of Obstetricians and Gynecologists has increased from about 10,000 in 1965 to more than 25,000 in 1985. Between 1975 and 1987, the average number of visits to Ob/Gyns declined from 104.2 per week to 88.2 per week. In a period when the supply of obstetricians exceeds the demand, Ob/Gyns may be inclined to pay more attention to other kinds of services. Moreover, some Ob/Gyns are drifting away from the practice of obstetrics because of concern over the rising cost of malpractice insurance, greater reluctance to be on-call at all hours, and a trend toward increasing specialization in medicine generally. [62]

Another factor that may have encouraged physicians to increase their attention to infertility is the increased prestige accorded the infertility specialty as a result of the publicity surrounding IVF and other high-tech treatments. The newer therapies for infertility—I include here clomiphene citrate, hMG, and the several variations of artificial insemination as well as IVF and GIFT—are cyclical or "continual" therapies that may be repeated if they do not succeed the first time; possible repetition may also contribute to the attractiveness of infertility treatment for physicians.[63]

Again I note here that the medicalization of infertility is primarily a middle-class phenomenon. Relatively well-off couples are increasingly seeking treatment for infertility. Blacks and those with lower incomes are not as likely to pursue infertility treatment. I argue in this book that the medicalization of infertility has had striking implications for the experience of infertility. In this context, the fact that my sample is made up of white, primarily middle-class couples appears more as an advantage than as a disadvantage. These are, after all, the couples we would expect to be most profoundly affected by the trend toward medicalization.

INFERTILITY AND THE MEDICAL MODEL

To say that infertility is becoming medicalized is to say that it is becoming seen as being like an illness. But even if infertility is viewed as an illness, it differs in several important ways from illness as the medical model typically conceives of it. Although illness is usually seen as a phenomenon affecting an individual, typically *couples* experience infertility. Regardless of which member of a couple has impaired fertility, it is the couple as a unit that is deprived of the experience of parenthood. Sociologist Barbara Katz Rothman points out, "For women, the single most common cause of infertility is . . . mating with an infertile man. (Conversely, the single most common cause of infertility in men is mating with an infertile woman.)"[64] As I discuss in succeeding chapters, individuals who do not have a diagnosed reproductive impairment may still think of themselves as infertile.

Although the proper medical focus in infertility treatment is on the couple, medical care of the wife in the early stages of treatment is seldom well coordinated with that of the husband. Women are treated by gynecologists or infertility specialists, men by urologists who may or may not specialize in infertility. Gynecologists refer to urologists, and vice-versa, but they seldom share a practice. Husbands rarely go with their wives to appointments with gynecologists; wives almost never accompany their husbands to the offices of urologists. Lack of coordination between medical treatment of wives and husbands complicates the treatment process for the couple.

Regardless of which member of the couple has the reproductive impairment, the female partner first displays symptoms: It is she who does not get pregnant. And, regardless of who has the reproductive impairment, the female partner is likely to be subjected to a series of painful and intrusive tests. An ironic feature of infertility treatment is that the person with the reproductive impairment is not necessarily the person treated. Even when the man is the only partner with a diagnosed reproductive impairment, the woman still may undergo invasive treatments. The most obvious case where this happens is with artificial insemination, but IVF and hMG are both routinely used in cases of male infertility as well as in cases of infertility without diagnosis.

This brings me to a second characteristic of infertility that distinguishes it from illness as typically understood by the medical model. Infertility is not really a pathological condition; rather, it is the absence of a desired condition. A couple with no physical symptoms— only their failure to have a desired child—is just as infertile as a couple in which one or both members has an obvious physiological impairment. Thus, it is theoretically impossible for an infertile couple to be diagnosed as normal. An infertile couple with no apparent pathological condition is still infertile; such a couple is described not as being normal but as having "idiopathic" infertility.

Because infertility is the absence of a desired condition rather than the presence of a pathological condition, it is for most couples an open-ended affair. Because the female reproductive process is cyclical, infertility is cyclical. Although there are some couples who literally have no chance for a pregnancy, for the vast majority infertility is something experienced one month at a time. At the same time that a woman's menstrual period brings disappointment it also announces that a new cycle is beginning.

A third difference between infertility and illness typically conceived is that infertility has solutions other than biological achievement of pregnancy. If infertility is the absence of a desired condition, then one possibility (theoretically, at least) is to stop desiring the condition. To put the matter more straightforwardly, a couple can choose to adopt or remain childless. Another obvious alternative to biological solutions is the pursuit of adoption. For most infertility specialists, the primary goal of treatment is a cure, that is, a pregnancy. Nonmedical solutions—such as adoption and childless living—are often viewed as options to be considered only when attempts at a normal pregnancy have proven futile.[65]

INFERTILITY AS A CHRONIC ILLNESS

If infertility is like an illness, then the kind of illness it is like is chronic illness. Chronic illnesses are characterized, not only by their long-term nature, but also by their inherent uncertainty and the extent to which they intrude on the lives of sufferers.[66] Some sources of infertility, such as endometriosis, are quite literally chronic illnesses. Others, such as tubal scarring, usually due to iatrogenic (medically induced) causes or to Pelvic Inflammatory Disease, are not chronic illnesses in the most literal sense of the term. For most cases of infertility, it may be more appropriate to speak in terms of an *analogy* between infertility and chronic illness rather than to speak of infertility as a *type* of chronic illness. To state it simply, being infertile is *like* having a chronic illness.

Although my sample may not be completely representative, a mean duration of from 5.2 years (husbands' estimates) to 6.7 years (wives' estimates) seems to qualify infertility as a long-term condition. In many types of chronic illness and disability, the demands of an invasive and extensive treatment regimen can assume such importance and make such demands on an individual's time and energy that they dwarf other interests and roles. As I discuss in Chapters 3 and 4, the infertile, like the chronically ill and disabled, also find that treatment regimens assume a central importance in their lives.

Treatment for infertility is often expensive, time-consuming, and invasive. For example, a frequently prescribed drug for ovulation problems is human menopausal gonadotropin (hMG), which costs about 700 dollars per monthly cycle. Administration of hMG requires daily injections and consistent monitoring of blood levels for the first half of each cycle as well as monthly sonograms. The wives in my sample had collectively undergone at least fourteen hysterosalpingograms, thirteen diagnostic surgeries, and seventeen major surgeries. The husbands in my sample had collectively undergone at least three surgeries and countless collections of semen for diagnostic purposes.

Two practices commonly recommended to infertile couples are the charting of basal body temperature (BBT) upon arising each morning and the scheduling of intercourse to maximize the likelihood of conception.[67] It does not take much imagination to see that these two practices are likely to constitute intrusions into everyday life that continually remind couples of their infertility. Thus, like the chronically ill, the infertile may come to feel that the quality of their lives has been adversely affected by their condition and that the treatment regimen now occupies an imposing place in their lives.

As in chronic illness, the experience of infertility is characterized by uncertainty in the illness trajectory of infertility.[68] While much of the uncertainty inherent in many chronic conditions revolves around the fear of relapse, the experience of uncertainty among the infertile is more likely to revolve around the hope for a miracle. New treatments are constantly being developed, and the possibility of new treatments is always being discussed. As I have already noted, approximately half the couples treated for infertility become pregnant, and treatment-independent pregnancies are quite common. For a number of reasons, few couples are ever told they have no chance to conceive. Although the source of uncertainty in infertility may be different from the source of uncertainty in chronic illness, the instability inherent in both conditions makes adjustment difficult.

If the analogy between infertility and chronic illness is apt, this may have as much to do with the ways in which infertility is defined and treated as with the nature of infertility as a physical condition. Many aspects of infertility that the people I spoke with complained about—the pervasive nature of treatment demands, the embarrassing aspects of certain tests, the uncertainty with regard to prognosis—are aimed as much at the treatment of their condition as at the condition itself. Given this observation, it seems reasonable to surmise that as medicalization progresses, infertility is becoming more like chronic illness than before.

THREE

BODIES AND SELVES
Infertility, Gender, and Identity

People often use mental timetables to assess their progress in a particular line of action. Such timetables are often guided by "age norms," socially approved standards for the timing of life events. Family historians have argued that transitions from one life stage to another in American society and other industrial societies have become more uniform and predictable in the twentieth century than they were previously.[1]

THE NORM OF PARENTHOOD

In American society, parenthood is seen as an integral part of the transition to adult status.[2] It is relatively easy to document that parenthood is regarded as normative and childlessness as deviant.[3] Studies of American women show that approximately 90 to 95 percent see childlessness as an undesirable state for themselves and others.[4] Now that unmarried cohabitation is more acceptable than it has been in the past, it is possible that marriage has become even more closely associated with the desire to have children.[5]

As sociologist Charlene Miall asserts, not simply parenthood, but *biological* parenthood, is defined as normal. In his book, *American*

Kinship, anthropologist David Schneider shows that American kinship terminology revolves around the assumption that blood ties bind kin together. Recent media coverage of adoptees who search for their "real" parents reinforces the image that a normal parent is one who gives birth to and raises a child.[6]

To say that norms in American culture define the achievement of biological parenthood as an integral part of the transition to adulthood is not merely to assert that these are ideas inside people's heads. I do not see norms as lessons learned in childhood and then existing as some sort of internal gyroscope that impels behavior for the rest of one's life. Rather, I take the view that norms as expectations for behavior are embedded in the structure of social interaction.[7] The normality of parenthood is not something learned once and for all but, rather, something continually relearned in the course of everyday life. The normality of parenthood is communicated and reasserted by the media's presentations that depict and define "families" as people with children. It is also reinforced by the mere fact that parenthood is statistically normal; as they interact with people in everyday life, individuals cannot help but observe that most people of a certain age seem to have children.

But, most important, the sense that being a parent is an integral part of adulthood is communicated through the rituals of daily interaction. In the United States, after meeting someone for the first time, What do you do for a living? is probably the first question asked. Are you married? is probably the second; if one answers the second question affirmatively, the third question is likely to be, Do you have any children? After a while, "no" can come to feel like the wrong answer.

Both the wives and the husbands I spoke to shared this cultural sense that having children was a normal and natural part of being an adult. Jim's expectations for his marital future were typical: "Basically, we figured that we'd start with two and go from there, that we'd be the all-American family." Given these widespread expectations, it is important to look at the different ways in which wives and husbands responded to their inability to proceed with their lives according to the culturally prescribed timetable.

INFERTILE WIVES: SPOILED IDENTITY

In keeping with the medical model (see Chapter 2), it is common for both the healthy and the ill to think of their bodies as machines.[8] A corollary of the notion that the body is a machine is the idea that the body is a *thing*, whose functioning and malfunctioning can be described in purely physical terms and without reference to such ephemeral notions as mind or spirit or self.

If the body is experienced as a machine, then it stands to reason that disease and other types of health problems are likely to be experienced as mechanical failures. When they were asked how infertility had affected them, many wives I interviewed said they felt as if their bodies had failed.[9] Karen described her feelings about herself and her body: "It doesn't mean I'm not a good person; it just means my body's not working." Karen was very careful to distinguish clearly between herself and her body, but she was virtually alone in doing so. Most other wives who spoke of body failure seemed to think of *both* themselves and their bodies as having failed. Lynn's words reveal that she sees her defective body, not as something she *has* but as something she *is:* "I would consider that I am subfertile and that I do need correction."

Barbara, too, used language that made it seem as though her sense of personhood was intertwined with her appreciation of herself as a well-functioning machine: "I had this feeling of failure, an overwhelming image of failure as a baby machine and as a woman." Thus, the majority of wives mixed their metaphors. At the same time that they saw their bodies as machines, they also identified their bodies with their selves so that their sense of themselves as viable persons seemed to depend on the sense of themselves as viable machines. Although the medical model may view health problems as merely physical conditions, it seems quite difficult for infertile wives to separate their bodies from themselves. They described themselves as having not only imperfect bodies but also *spoiled identities*.[10]

Many infertile wives I talked with described themselves as feeling inadequate as women. Debby characterized herself as "feeling real,

real defective."[11] Rachel put it this way: "I felt not as good as any-body else. You know, like everybody else can get pregnant, and I can't."

Wives' sense of failure was not limited to the sphere of reproduction alone. For many wives, the sense of being a failure spilled over to contaminate all facets of identity. Debby elaborated on the way infertility affected her sense of self:

> It affects your ego. It has an immense effect on self-concept, in all kinds of crazy ways. You ask "How can I be a real woman?" By affecting the self-concept, it affects sexuality, and it affected work for me for a while. "How can I be good at this; I'm not a normal person."

A number of the wives I interviewed described themselves as feeling incomplete. Peg said, "Sometimes I felt that I wasn't really a whole person." Mary used death imagery to describe her sense of failure and incompleteness:

> It was as if a part of me had died, a part of me was never going to be fulfilled. Grieving to hold a baby. A part of me felt like I was never going to be, a part of me felt like a major disappointment to everybody. I think that was the hardest thing. I felt like I had disappointed my husband, I disappointed my folks, I disappointed his folks, and I disappointed myself.

Martha employed the language of disability to express her sense of incompleteness: "A lot of times I've felt I'm not a complete woman. I've often thought of it as being similar to being handicapped."

Why are these women so willing to accept personal responsibility for a situation that seems, on the face of it, outside their control? Social psychologist Melvin Lerner posits that people need to believe in a just world in which people are punished for misdeeds and rewarded for proper behavior.[12] Such a belief, Lerner argues, leads people—under certain conditions, at any rate—to hold those who appear to be innocent victims of circumstances beyond their control as ultimately responsible for their own plight. The belief in a just world is so strong, Lerner argues, that innocent victims even tend to devalue themselves.

Whether or not the tendency to blame the victim is part of human nature, as Lerner seems to suggest, it seems to me that this tendency serves some important social control functions as well. Social groups are always on the lookout for ways to enforce norms held to be important. Any undesired state of affairs—infertility, blindness, epilepsy, leprosy—can be seized upon as a sanction against taboo behavior. The stigmatization of sufferers as people who deserve their fate is merely a by-product of this social control mechanism. Because sufferers, too, have been socialized to accept cultural values, they may share the view that sufferers are personally responsible for their own misfortune.[13] (I develop these ideas further in Chapter 7.)

Let us look for a moment at the words Lois used to describe the way infertility affected her sense of self: "I never felt much like a woman, so to speak. I just felt like I was useless. Which is ridiculous. I know that, but there were times I felt like that." Lois seems confused. She knows that infertility is not her fault, but still she feels like a failure. She has internalized not only the societal definition that fertility is the normal state of affairs, but also the socially instilled judgment that people who suffer must be somehow inferior. In spite of her own better judgment, she finds it hard not to think of herself as personally responsible for her own infertility.

One must not assume that the wives I am describing here are more traditional than other American women or that they have somehow escaped the influence of the ideological and social changes of the past several decades. During my interview with Teri, she described herself as a feminist. Later in the interview, I asked her how she reconciled her feminism with her strong desire for motherhood. She responded, "It makes me feel confused, you know, because I'm a little surprised at how I've taken all this. Because the way that I was, I wouldn't have thought that it would have thrown me for such a loop."

INFERTILE HUSBANDS: A BAD BREAK

Although few data have been collected on the question of men's and women's reactions to infertility, what little evidence there is suggests that, just as his marriage is better than hers, so seemingly his infertility is better than hers.[14]

My interviews, too, indicate that wives were more likely than husbands to see infertility as a devastating experience. Of the wives I interviewed, nineteen (including all but one wife with no diagnosed reproductive impairment) felt that infertility had personally affected them a great deal, but only nine husbands agreed. Of the husbands I interviewed, twelve (including five of the ten with a diagnosed reproductive impairment and all three with no diagnosis) felt that infertility had affected them only slightly or not at all. No wife could agree.

Husbands were less likely to speak in terms that would lead us to believe they saw themselves as having spoiled identities. A few husbands, however, did use the language of body failure. According to Dan, "To find out there's a part of me that doesn't work right was just crushing." And Rick used words reminiscent of those used by many wives: "I didn't feel like I was a complete man at the time."

It is interesting to note that only husbands who themselves had a reproductive impairment described themselves as having spoiled identities.[15] Wives, however, were likely to see themselves in terms of spoiled identity regardless of whether they themselves had a reproductive impairment.

The majority of husbands viewed the experience of infertility as disappointing but not devastating. Earlier, I quoted Teri, the "feminist" who reported being "thrown for a loop"; her husband Jeff described his quite different feelings: "It's not the end of the world at all. I don't rate this up there as one of the tragedies of all time." Jim spoke in similar terms: "My own personal problem with infertility— basically, it didn't exist. I pursued the why and the wherefore of it to see if it could be fixed. If it could, great, but I wasn't a goner if it couldn't be fixed."

These husbands tended to be fatalistic about infertility, seeing it as something they could get over if they had to. As Lee put it, "I guess I always kind of felt whatever happens, happens, and I'll just go ahead with the treat..ents. If it works, it works. If it doesn't, it doesn't." Dave had a similar attitude: "If you determine that you want to have kids, you do everything you can to accomplish a goal. And if you've done everything you can and you still can't, then you should accept it and go on."

These husbands, however, are clearly neither oblivious nor insensitive to the way their wives are reacting to infertility. Peter, aware of how his wife Kim felt and of how she expected him to feel, expressed confusion over the fact that he didn't feel that way:

> My personal infertility has never tormented me. I've sometimes wondered if I have some sort of mental problem or something that it hasn't. It's never really eaten away at me. Maybe I've just permanently flipped the switch to think about other things or something like that. Maybe subconsciously I am tormented, but I've talked myself out of feeling tormented or something. I don't know, but I just don't feel that sorry for myself.

CONFRONTING THE FERTILE WORLD

Perhaps because they experienced infertility as a catastrophic role failure, most wives reported that infertility came to permeate every aspect of their lives. Infertility was something they always thought about and could never escape. Infertility, in other words, became a "master status."[16]

To use Debby's words, the infertile wives in my sample saw the world as a "fertile village," full of reminders that the rest of the world assumed parenthood was both normal and easy to achieve. For these wives, the routine interactions of everyday life continually reinforced their sense of failure and isolation. Pregnant women and babies were, for wives, constant and ubiquitous reminders of their inadequacy. A brief excerpt from my interview with Janet is illustrative:

Interviewer: Is being infertile something you'd say you think of once in a while or something you think of constantly?

Janet: Subconsciously, I think it's a lot more than I realize, but I think a lot.

Interviewer: Would you say that you ever go through a day without thinking about it?

Janet: Uh Uh. No, because I always see somebody that's pregnant or always somebody that's got a little baby, just wishing it was me instead of them.

According to Peg, "Every time that I'd see a pregnant woman, I'd just stare at her stomach. And holding babies would start getting to me."

One might think that infertile wives would see work as a refuge from infertility, a place where they could get their minds off reproduction and concentrate on something else, a source of a different kind of gratification that could at least partially compensate for the pain of infertility. My quantitative research with 449 infertile couples showed that employment did not reduce levels of worry about various spheres of everyday life for involuntarily childless women. Studies by a group of researchers at Pennsylvania State University are equivocal about whether involuntary childlessness affected job satisfaction among a sample of older rural women.[17] On the basis of my interviews, I think it is safe to say that—at this stage of their lives, at any rate—these infertile wives did not find in work an alternate source of gratification, a compensation for the suffering caused by infertility.

On the contrary, many wives I interviewed saw work as just one more place in which to be reminded of infertility. Mary found it difficult to be at work because she encountered so many reminders of her infertility there:

Work became real tough. Having to go into work and be a manager and leave my personal feelings at home and always be on top of things when in the back of my mind I was always thinking about something else. Having to manage pregnant women was real tough. Being sympathetic when they had to go home early because they got sick—I didn't really care.

Cindy also found work full of reminders of infertility: "Work was very hard for me because there were a lot of pregnant women at work. A lot of them. There were three a year. They had baby showers right there at work, and that bothered me. I don't think people understood how upset I was. They had a Christmas party and they wanted everyone to bring his baby pictures. [laughter] I did not go. As a matter of fact, I called in sick." And Robin changed jobs; she chose to work in an all-male office where she wouldn't be confronted by baby showers.

One might think that a church or a synagogue would be one place that might provide infertile wives with a refuge from feelings of failure, incompleteness, and loneliness. And, indeed a few wives did find some comfort in the social support they received in church. Both Lois and Kate said that the people they knew from church were supportive and that their support was helpful. They were, however, outnumbered by those who saw religious organizations as one more obstacle to be overcome in their struggle to cope with infertility. The recurrent theme sounded by these wives was that church is a family-centered institution, frequented by pregnant women and young children, where one cannot help but be reminded of one's own infertile status. Cathy described a brief experiment with church attendance: "I thought, 'Well, I think I better go to church.' Maybe in going to church and listening to sermons and things, I'll find some answers. At least it would give me time to meditate. God, that is the worst place to go if you're infertile."

Many wives spoke of emotional difficulties they encountered in other public places. Sally talked of her feelings about grocery stores: "They sometimes just drive me wild. I swear, every woman I see is either pregnant or has a baby in the cart. And I'm dashing down aisles, you know, hoping old people are around the bend." Jean found toy stores hard to deal with: "It was really hard whenever there was an occasion to buy a gift for a child of a friend or a relative. It was really hard to go into a store and deal with that. A lot of times we would order things through catalogues rather than dealing with going into a toy store." Carol was bothered by bookstores: "For the last couple years, I've been looking for adoption titles or child care titles or things like that. And there are eight zillion books on pregnancy. For some reason, that just gets my dander up. I don't know why. Maybe that's where all my hostility is coming out. I want to take a match to them."

The events these wives describe might seem innocuous to the fertile reader; they are merely routine events of everyday life. Unlike the chronically ill or disabled, the infertile wives I interviewed have not been physically prevented from attending or enjoying these activities. Instead, these normal activities have become unbearable because they dramatize for the infertile wife her sense that she has been denied access to normality.

Reminders of infertility are not limited to public places. Thanks to television, the fertile world can penetrate the privacy of one's home. Jean said that she was particularly bothered by diaper commercials. Kate was troubled not so much by the commercials as by the regular programming: "Sometimes, if I would see a television program about families, I'd get angry and think, 'Why isn't my family like that family?'"

Painful reminders of infertility also enter the home by means of the treatment regimen itself (I expand upon this point in Chapter 4). Infertile wives find that their regimens often assume a central importance in their lives. Two wives described some ways in which the subtle but continual demands of the treatment regimen imposed themselves on their outlooks. Karen said that she thought about infertility every day: "I have to deal with it every moment of my life. All the people we have at work who are pregnant. And every day I have to look at the calendar and see what day of the cycle it is and see whether it's a pill day or a sex day or whatever. I mean, I have to live with this every day of my life." Robin also spoke of constantly encountering reminders of infertility:

It was an everyday thing. Because you have to take your temperature every morning and when you have to take your temperature every morning, it's hard not to think about why you're taking your temperature. And everything anybody said to me, I could always relate it to being infertile. I was more sensitive. People could say something to me that maybe a year or so before would never have affected me, and now I would just run outside to cry.

Four husbands, three of whom themselves had reproductive impairments, shared with their wives the sense that they were surrounded by a fertile world. Dan, who had a low sperm count, described his difficulties at work: "I'm a school psychologist who works with little kids, seeing parents every day and doing therapy with people who have fucked-up families and who don't seem to give a damn about their kids. It affects me every day. It still does. It affects me daily." Rick discussed the reasons he and his wife stopped going to church: "In the beginning, we would go to church a lot. It was one escape. It helped, but then, all of a sudden, it seemed like everybody was pregnant. Then we couldn't handle it anymore."

But, in general, husbands were much less likely to see infertility as something pervasive from which it was impossible to escape. While nineteen wives (including six of the seven who did not have a diagnosed reproductive impairment) reported thinking about infertility virtually "all the time," only eight husbands reported being preoccupied with it, although this number does include five of the ten husbands with diagnosed reproductive impairments. Husbands were less likely to avoid child-centered activities or to feel that infertility was something inescapable. Tom described his strategy for putting infertility out of his mind: "I feel I can keep myself going by immersing myself in other things. Work was the big one for awhile. I play guitar, and I go in stages where I pull a guitar out and play madly for a period of time, and then I put it away again. I've been very active in sports, through work and outside of work." Lee, too, claimed he found it relatively easy to immerse himself in other things, but he denied that this was a strategy for dealing with infertility:

> Well, I don't think I've really done anything much different than I did prior to our infertility problems. I still enjoy golf and tennis and bowling and a lot of activities that I've enjoyed right along. If it really bothered me a lot, I think I would probably get more involved in other things. I keep myself very busy with projects around the house and other things, but I don't think I'm busier than ever before, and I don't do it to keep my mind off it because my mind isn't really on it that much.

Dave's attitude toward infertility was typical of that of many husbands: "I'd say it's always in the background of my life, but I don't think about it that much because I don't waste my time thinking about things that are out of my control."

While two husbands seemed oblivious to the fact that their wives felt tormented by intrusions of the fertile world into their lives, most husbands were quite aware that their wives were distressed by the sight of pregnant women, children, and other reminders of their infertility. A few husbands seemed on occasion to get upset at intrusions from the fertile world, not so much on their own account, but rather on behalf of their wives. Stuart, who has remained very active in his church, described an incident that he and his wife Lois found upsetting:

> One time at church on Mother's Day, the minister asked all the children to go around and hug all the women that didn't have children in church. And after church, Lois just broke down crying. You know, we didn't want children to come over and hug us, to remind us that we can't have children. And the

62

following Mother's Day we didn't go to that service. We refused
to go.

Thus, husbands were not only less likely than their wives to see infertility as a threat to identity, but they were also less likely to see
themselves as living in a world where painful reminders of infertility
were inescapable.

GENDER AND THE EXPERIENCE OF INFERTILITY

There are several possible explanations for gender differences in the
experience of infertility. First, I must consider the possibility that
the differences I purport to uncover may be more apparent than real.
Perhaps husbands were simply less likely than wives to reveal their
feelings to the interviewers. A substantial body of literature testifies
to the fact that men are typically less willing than women to make
self-disclosures with regard to intimate or personal matters.[18] Furthermore, all husbands were interviewed by male interviewers; possibly husbands were unwilling to admit feelings of inadequacy and
failure in front of other men.

The social dynamics of the interviewing situation itself inevitably
differ for husbands and wives, but I am not inclined to think that the
gender differences I have found are *merely* artifacts of gender differences in interview dynamics. Husbands did, in fact, make many self-
threatening disclosures. Any reader of my transcripts would, I
think, be impressed with how frank both husbands and wives are in
their discussions of very sensitive themes, such as sexuality. In fact, a
husband's admission to an interviewer that infertility is "not such a
big deal" can be seen as a bold and risky disclosure if his wife thinks
infertility is indeed a big deal and assumes he thinks so too.

Still, we must not discount the possibility that some differences
between husbands and wives that I have described may stem from
the fact that, in American society, different "feeling rules" apply to

men and women.[19] In other words, men and women are subject to different expectations about what emotions they will (and should) experience and how (and whether) they will (and should) express these emotions. Thus, women are depicted in popular media as being more emotionally expressive than men; and evidence suggests that women and men identify with and conform to these expectations. Since the nineteenth century, the idea that wives are emotional specialists and that husbands are instrumental specialists has been influential in American society. Although the power of the "doctrine of the two spheres" has lost power in recent years, Lillian Rubin has shown that the division of couples into expressive wives and inexpressive husbands is still a reality in many American marriages.[20] Perhaps my data represent—at least in part—one more contemporary enactment of this long-standing sexual script.

Second, and also related to the two spheres, I consider the process of industrialization and the concomitant separation of paid work from domestic life. As Cancian points out, the "feminization of love" in the nineteenth century developed alongside the "masculinization of work." In the American family myth, husbands have been more closely identified with the roles of breadwinner, protector, and provider, while wives have been more closely associated with the roles of nurturer and caretaker. Again, Lillian Rubin provides convincing evidence that this myth is still a powerful psychological reality.[21]

I have suggested that a major source of the identity consequences of infertility is an inability to conform to the age norms the individual has internalized. Parenthood is normative for both husbands and wives, but the parent role is more central to the transition to adulthood for women than for men. There is, in American society, no "fatherhood mandate" with the same force and intensity as the "motherhood mandate."[22] Because parenthood is deemed more central to women's identity than to men's, then the effects of infertility on identity are arguably more severe for women than for men.

Third, wives probably *are* exposed to more reminders of infertility during the course of their daily activities.[23] Wives are more likely than their husbands to be employed in positions where they come into frequent contact with children. They are also more likely than their husbands to work around other women, who can be expected to converse about pregnancy, childbirth, and children more often than men do. And, outside work, they are more likely to find themselves in the company of other women—at baby showers, aerobics classes, volunteer activities, and so forth—where children and pregnancy are common subjects of conversation.

Wives, more likely to do the shopping for their families, are therefore more likely to be in the toy stores and supermarkets that the infertile wives I spoke with found so crammed with reminders of their infertility. Wherever wives go, they are much more likely to be asked about their families. And the people they meet are more likely to assume that they have an interest in hearing detailed accounts of children, pregnancy, and delivery. Thus, women's daily round of life reinforces the notion that parenthood *ought* to be central to their identities.

Fourth, regardless of who, if anyone, has the reproductive impairment, it is the wife who fails to become pregnant. Thus, the biological drama of infertility—the roller-coaster cycle of hopefulness followed by the disastrous emotional letdown that comes with the beginning of each period—is played out in the wife's body. Regardless of who is biologically "at fault," it is the wife who is unable to display the visible signs of an expected and desired change in status.

The fact that husbands who themselves had reproductive impairments were considerably more likely than husbands without reproductive impairments to have "female" reactions to infertility suggests that the actual experience of body failure is a key aspect of suffering a spoiled identity. But a major difference exists between husbands and wives: for husbands, but not wives, the experience of body failure is limited to those with reproductive impairments.

Fifth, at least some effects I have described may concern the treatment regimen involved in infertility as much as they involve the infertile state itself. For example, such reminders of infertility as BBT charts and medication schedules are part of the treatment regimen and would be avoided if treatment were not being pursued. If the medicalization of infertility is in part responsible for the identity consequences of infertility, then we should expect these consequences to be more pronounced for wives than for husbands because the lives of the wives have been more profoundly affected by medicalization. After all, the wife must take her BBT every morning, and her blood levels are those monitored. Even if the husband has the reproductive impairment, the wife is still the focus of artificial insemination or IVF. Remember, the wives in my sample had, as a group, undergone thirty surgical procedures compared to three for their husbands. And remember that, while office visits for infertility have increased dramatically in recent years among women, men's visits have remained at virtually the same level as before.[24]

I must point out here that I interviewed middle-class couples. Because treatment seeking is related to class status, it is likely that the medicalization of infertility has proceeded further among middle-class women than it has among lower- and working-class women, a trend reflected in other areas of reproductive health.[25] We might speculate that, because middle-class women are not as accustomed as working-class women to being unable to realize their ambitions, middle-class women might experience the failure of infertility more acutely. Feelings of failure might also be stronger among middle-class women because poor and minority women often have kin-based networks that provide opportunities for informal adoption and childkeeping, options not as available to white, middle-class women.[26] Middle-class men, however, might be expected to be less affected by infertility than working-class men. Virility seems a more important theme in the culture of working-class males than in that of middle-class males, and having a biological child may be seen as proof of that virility.[27] For the present, it is clearly impossible to generalize from my sample to members of other social classes.

The reader will have noted by now that I have not attributed the differences in wives' and husbands' responses to infertility to innate differences between men and women. Questions of whether maternal instincts exist and how genetic influences may affect differences in behavior between men and women have been the subject of much research and even more debate. It is beyond the scope of this book to attempt to resolve the "nature vs. nurture" question. Whatever the influence of genes on human behavior, I do not think that reference to innate differences between men and women goes far to explain why, in contemporary America, infertile wives seem more distressed by infertility than their husbands.

My chief reason for not giving much credence to innate differences as an explanation for differing responses to infertility is that the meaning of children, and therefore the meaning of infertility, varies both crossculturally and historically. If the differences I have observed between infertile wives and their husbands were due primarily to innate differences between men and women, then we would expect husbands to react similarly in all cultures and in all historical epochs. But this does not appear to be the case: That many cultures allow the husband of a childless wife to divorce her and remarry or to take a second wife (see Chapter 1) indicates that the men of some cultures are apparently much less willing to take infertility in stride than many American men seem to be.

Differing degrees of husband investment in having children are apparently related to differences in the meaning and value of children, which are in turn related to social and economic differences between societies. In many societies, the husband's strong interest in having children (usually sons) is related to the need to have a material and spiritual heir.[28] In other societies, where needing an heir is less of a factor, children are still valued for the economic assistance they can provide to the family and for the support they can provide in old age.

In contemporary American society, children are not valued so much for the material assistance or the family continuity they can provide as for the companionship and affection they are thought to supply. Lois Hoffman and Jean Manis asked a national probability sample of 2,025 married women and men an open-ended question about what they perceived to be the advantages of having children.

The most popular responses were those that had to do with primary group ties and affection; 65.8 percent of white women and 59.5 percent of white men volunteered these kinds of responses. Only 4.0 percent of white women and 3.1 percent of white men mentioned economic reasons for valuing children. Reasons mentioning continuity of family or self were given by 4.0 percent of white women and 16.2 percent of white men.[29]

In contemporary American society, men are probably less concerned with having an heir than they may once have been, because, except for the very wealthy, most people do not have appreciable fixed property to pass on. Furthermore, the development of the importance of educational credentials as a means of validating social and economic status has meant that the possession of wealth, though it still greatly enhances one's ability to get one's children established, is no guarantee that one's stature in society can be extended beyond one's own lifetime.[30] Thus, children may be more a source of status anxiety than a symbol of the permanence of one's place in life. And, far from being seen as economic assets, children are far more often viewed as expensive propositions, only justifiable in noneconomic terms.

In *Pricing the Priceless Child*, Viviana Zelizer traces the process in American society during the period from 1870 through 1930 by which the "useful" child, valued for the labor and support he or she could offer, was replaced by the "useless" child, valued for nontangible benefits, such as warmth and affection.[31] Zelizer argues that, as labor moved from the home to the factory and as the family's locus moved from production to intimacy, children came to be valued—first by the middle class and later by the working class—as functionally worthless but emotionally priceless beings.

Because the developing idea of two spheres defined affection and emotion as primarily women's sphere,[32] this transvaluation of childhood may have effectively decreased men's investment in children. If it is true that men's concerns about having children have traditionally focused on issues of heirship and economic usefulness, then perhaps one by-product of the "sacralization of childhood" was a certain degree of "feminization" of the desire to procreate.[33]

These last remarks are admittedly speculative. I have no evidence to prove why it is that infertile husbands in contemporary America seem to have less of an investment in procreation than their wives. But, for my present purposes, it is not necessary for me to prove that I can explain this phenomenon once and for all. My goal here is simply to convince the reader that the explanation probably lies not in the domain of invariant human nature, but rather in changes in social structure and ideology.

On the face of it, the evidence I have presented here to the effect that infertile wives are more affected by infertility than their husbands seems to contradict the assertion by some critics of reproductive technology that men are more committed to biological parenthood than women and that women often resort to these technologies under pressure from their husbands.[34] Judith Lasker and Susan Borg suggest that men are more committed than women to biological parenthood because their main contribution to a child is genetic; they therefore are more concerned than women with carrying on the family name and heritage. Michelle Stanworth asserts that, because women bear children and generally take primary responsibility for rearing them, men may be insecure about the basis for a relationship with a child not genetically linked to them.[35]

Several studies of people who have had recourse to the new reproductive technologies have found some evidence that infertile wives sometimes feel pressured by their husbands to continue to try to have a biological child when they themselves would be content to adopt.[36] The advent of the use of IVF in the treatment of male reproductive impairments offers a particularly strong challenge to my picture of husbands' and wives' reactions to infertility. From the wife's point of view, artificial insemination by donor (AID) might seem the preferable option in cases where there is no female reproductive impairment because it would achieve the same effect—pregnancy—without requiring surgery. After all, one might argue, if women are so much more disturbed by infertility than men, why would couples choose to pursue IVF rather than the much simpler and less invasive procedure of AID?

The difference between my findings and those obtained in the studies to which I have just referred may have something to do with differences in the characteristics of the samples studied. The studies just mentioned all focused on women or couples who were actively pursuing IVF, surrogate motherhood, or some other of the new reproductive "technologies." Thus, it might be argued that these studies concentrated on those most committed to biological parenthood. Most couples in my sample, however, had either decided against IVF or never considered it, none had ever considered surrogate motherhood, and only a few had pursued AID. While the studies alluded to above may have oversampled couples where husbands were committed to biological parenthood, I may have undersampled those couples.

In any case, the willingness of wives to undergo IVF or other procedures for the sake of their husbands does not necessarily contradict my findings that wives' identities are more contaminated by infertility than are those of their husbands. If a wife were motivated to do whatever it takes to have a baby and if her less motivated husband preferred childlessness to adopting a baby that was not "really" his, then opting for IVF, surrogate motherhood, or other less conventional options might seem like a natural solution. Lorber refers to such instances where a wife goes along with her husband's wishes to preserve peace in the family as "patriarchal bargains."[37] Further research, of course, is necessary to determine whether such negotiations actually occur in the case of infertility.

But even if a woman's spouse is not the source of the pressure to escape from infertility by whatever means necessary, that does not mean that there is not still considerable pressure to pursue infertility treatment.[38] In my sample, the main source of pressure on infertile wives to pursue treatment came, not from husbands or any other specific people, but from their acceptance of norms about what it means to be an adult in American society, from their sense that they had failed to live up to these norms, and from the reminders of both these norms and their failures that were ever-present in their contacts with the fertile world.

In this chapter I have tried to demonstrate that such pressures are powerful indeed. The effects of infertility on identity differ for wives and husbands; given the differences in the ways wives and husbands experience infertility, they understandably have different responses to infertility treatment.

FOUR

IMPATIENT PATIENTS
Negotiating Infertility Treatment

Ａs we saw in Chapter 3, the wives and husbands I interviewed shared with most Americans the expectation that they would be parents. Robin's comments plainly reveal that she had regarded parenthood as something so easy to achieve that it could be easily taken for granted: "Okay, I wanted four, he wanted two, so I figured we'd have two and an accident."

DISCOVERING INFERTILITY

A few people I spoke with did suspect that their reproductive capacities might be impaired. Dee, Rachel, and Mary knew they were DES daughters; therefore, they were aware that it might be hard for them to conceive. Debby learned soon after her marriage to Richard that she had endometriosis. Craig and Dave knew before they married their present wives that they were likely to have difficulty fathering a child. Cathy said she had a vague suspicion that she might have a hard time becoming pregnant even though she could not recall a concrete basis for her fears.

But the vast majority of both husbands and wives were taken by total surprise when they became aware of their infertility. Cathy's husband Chip had no inkling that fertility would be a problem: "I mean, when I think back now, I realize how dumb I really was. The word 'infertility' never even meant anything to me. I mean, I don't think I ever heard it." When I asked Teri if she ever suspected that it would be hard for her to conceive, she replied:

> I was thinking just the opposite. I was taking birth control pills for the first year after we got married. I remember one day, I got halfway to work, and I realized that I had forgotten to take my pill. Now, I could have taken it in the afternoon when I got home, but I was so paranoid that I'd get pregnant that I turned around and drove all the way home to take my pill. So that's how sure I was that just the opposite would be true.

The realization that there was indeed an infertility problem often occasioned a corresponding sense of "loss of control." Cathy was shocked to learn that she wasn't in control of her body: "I guess loss of control is going to have to come in here. That I didn't have any control over my destiny. It was a real shock to me to find something that I couldn't do anything about."

A number of writers on infertility have noted that this sense of lost control is common among the infertile.[1] The loss of control theme is especially important in understanding infertile wives' experience because the middle-class women in my sample had believed that they had control. In Chapter 2 I discussed the widespread use of birth control technology in the 1950s and 1960s, an important stage in the medicalization of reproduction. The people I interviewed are members of a group that has had a high degree of access to and confidence in birth control technology. They grew up believing that the human reproductive process is readily subject to human control.[2] As Lynn put it, "I thought having children would happen when we decided we were going to have them." These wives were surprised and demoralized when they realized that birth isn't quite as controllable as they had thought. Karen found irony in the fact that she had spent so many years practicing contraception before learning how difficult it would be for her to conceive: "If I'd known that we were going to have this problem, we never would have spent years on birth control."

If we think about it for a moment, we can see that infertile wives' sense of lost control may be related to the medical image of the body as machine. Machines, after all, can be manipulated by their operators. When machines malfunction, operators try to fix them. If they can't fix them, they feel helpless and out of control.

The couples I spoke with did find plausibility in the medical interpretation of infertility. They saw infertility as an organic problem susceptible to a technical solution. It is not surprising, then, that they turned to medical treatment as the most promising means of regaining a sense of control.[3] Sherry was explicit in linking her energetic pursuit of treatment to her desire to regain a sense of control. She tried to explain why she, not her husband Dan, took the lead in the treatment process: "Dan is more like, 'If I don't talk about it or think about it, it will go away.' And I'm the type that wants to know everything and feel as educated and as much in control of what I can control as possible. And, so I think that's why I'm the one to take charge."

In all twenty-two couples, the wife brought the issue of infertility up for discussion.[4] The wife's suspicion that there was a reproductive problem developed over a period of months during which she continued to have periods even though she had discontinued using contraception. Her recurring periods presented the physiological signal that something might be amiss.

While physicians typically do not consider a couple infertile until they have gone for at least a year of unprotected intercourse without conceiving, more than half the wives in my sample began to entertain seriously the belief that there was a problem well before a year had passed. This group includes all but one of those who suspected beforehand that they might have difficulty. The fact that a number of wives began to have serious concerns after only several months of unprotected intercourse attests to the power of the "motherhood mandate" in American society. Teri became convinced she was infertile after four months of trying when she lost a bet she had made with a friend over which of them would become pregnant first. Unlike Teri, most wives could not pinpoint a specific time or event when they began to see themselves as infertile. Rather they described the sense of themselves as infertile as something that crept up upon them day by day.

Wives shared their concerns with their husbands, who often tried to reassure them that everything was all right. Cathy described her early discussions with Chip about whether to pursue treatment:

> Initially, he would not admit that there was a problem. I felt really sure that there was a definite problem. Until they found something, there wasn't a problem in his mind. In my mind, we weren't pregnant, and we should have been by now so that's a problem. And he would not say that we were infertile for a long, long time, and I did. You know, I'd say, "We're not pregnant and we should have been by now, so we have a fertility problem." And he would say, "No, it's just taking us longer." I think that was a very frustrating time for me.

In twenty-one of twenty-two cases, the wife first presented herself to a physician for diagnosis and treatment. In one case the husband went for treatment: Jeff did so at Teri's suggestion; she had decided on the basis of her reading that this would be the best course of action because male reproductive impairments are easier to diagnose.

Most wives first mentioned their concerns to their regular gynecologists. Most wives broached the subject of infertility with their gynecologists during appointments scheduled for other purposes. In many cases, according to wives' accounts, gynecologists responded with assurance that there was nothing to worry about. Robin's gynecologist was confident that her fears were unfounded: "I mentioned it to my gynecologist, who said, 'Oh, no, there's nothing wrong.' He sent me on my way and said, 'See you in a year.' He said it was okay because my uterus was in the right place, and my Fallopian tubes felt good, and my ovaries were there. [Chuckle]. So, nope,

no problem" Janet's doctor advised her to relax: "He was a grand-
fatherly type, and he kept saying to me, 'Honey, you're just worrying too much. Go home and have yourself a couple of drinks and
relax.'"

It often took six months to a year or even longer for a woman and
her gynecologist to agree to define her as infertile. We have seen physicians' timetables differ from wives' timetables: wives typically
suspect the existence of a reproductive impairment sooner than physicians are willing to take their concerns seriously.[5] Physicians often
resisted wives' attempts to be recognized as infertile before the passage of what they felt was a suitable period of time. My data here
clearly support Catherine Kohler Riessman's argument that women
often participate actively in the process of medicalization.[6] Wives
sometimes had to broach the subject on several different occasions
before their gynecologists concurred that their difficulty conceiving
was a medical problem worth looking into. Jean described her attempt to prod her gynecologist into reluctantly beginning an infertility workup:

> After trying for about six months, I questioned my doctor,
> and he gave me a little slip of paper about relaxing and said to
> come back in six months. So I didn't really worry about it too
> much. Then, after six more months, I went back again. He gave
> me basal body temperature charts and told me to do that for
> three months and then to come back. So we did that for three
> months. When I came back, he said that everything looked
> good to him, and he sent me home. It was in the fall at that time
> and he said, "Come back in the spring, and you'll be pregnant."
> When I went back in the spring and nothing had happened, he
> told me that he would do an endometrial biopsy and sent Rick
> to a urologist.

What we observe here is, in fact, a process of negotiation; it is interesting both because it stretches over such a long period of time and also
because one negotiator so clearly controls the situation. Jean made a

claim to be deserving of treatment, but her doctor resisted her claim until she had persisted over a stretch of approximately fifteen months.[7] For most wives, then, validating their sense of themselves as infertile was a result of a long period of negotiations with physicians.

It is apparent from these comments that wives engineered couples' entry into infertility treatment. Throughout the treatment process, wives were more oriented toward treatment, regardless of who had the reproductive impairment. For example, wives usually proposed new treatment options for discussion. Lee put it succinctly: "I just went along with whatever had to be done. I never took the lead." According to Chip, Cathy took the leadership role in their discussions of treatment decisions:

> She was the leader. She made the moves. She'd say, "Well, I think we should do this now." And I'd say, "Okay, what does that mean?" And so we'd talk about it. It wasn't my idea to say, "Okay, let's go for a laparoscopy." It wasn't my idea to say, "Oh, let's do IVF." She kind of led me through the process.

Because (as we have seen in Chapter 3), infertility had a greater impact on identity for the wives in my sample, it should not surprise us that wives were much more oriented toward seeking treatment than their husbands. For wives, infertility presented itself as intolerable, identity-threatening; they were willing to do whatever it took to get out of it. Husbands often saw infertility as an unfortunate event that was to be put in perspective and then accepted.

PATIENT STRATEGIES

When infertile wives and their husbands enter the medical system, they become patients.[8] To become a patient means more than simply becoming the recipient of medical treatment; it also means becoming subjected to the expectations that comprise the patient role. Patients are expected to be the passive partners in the medical encounter.

They are expected to place themselves in the hands of physicians, letting them control the pace, tenor, and content of the medical interview. From the point of view of most physicians, a good patient is one who is compliant—that is, one who obeys doctors' orders.[9]

As medical sociologist Eliot Freidson has pointed out, interaction between doctors and patients is characterized by a power imbalance. Doctors have greater control than do patients over the direction and outcome of the medical interview. Studies of language use in the medical encounter have documented some strategies physicians employ to exercise control over the course of social interaction. In the typical medical interview, doctors give instructions *to* patients but seldom ask for instructions *from* patients. Doctors ask more questions of patients than patients ask of doctors, and they interrupt patients much more often than patients interrupt them. Because American medicine has historically embraced a view of women as more passive and less intellectually able than men, the power imbalance is even greater when the patient is a woman. Not surprisingly, given this power imbalance, patients are often dissatisfied with their physicians. Medical sociologist David Mechanic found that one-third of the people in one community reported that they had changed physicians owing to dissatisfaction.[10]

Thus, when infertile wives and husbands decide to seek medical treatment for infertility, they place themselves in a paradoxical situation, because—to regain a sense of control—they have found it necessary to place themselves in a situation where they have very little control indeed. The decision to take action to change their situation requires assuming a role in which they are expected to be passive. Relationships between infertile patients and their physicians are thus characterized by a latent conflict centering around the issue of control. We have already observed the first manifestation of this latent conflict: the infertile wife's first attempt to attract medical attention to her problem often involved a skirmish over the question of whose standards were to be used in defining the wife as infertile.

Because of the inherent power imbalance between doctors and patients, studies of medical encounters often characterize patients as passive reactors who have no choice but to acquiesce to doctors' control over the situation. But to say that patients have less power than doctors is not to say they lack power resources. To say patients have been cast in a passive role is not to say they always accept without question the part in which they have been cast. Patients may still use the resources available to them in their attempts to assert some control over the situation. [11]

Although most social scientific studies of encounters between doctors and patients seem to rest on the assumption that patients are passive, some studies of doctor-patient interaction assert that patients are in fact active agents attempting to assert control over a situation in which they lack power. Most of these studies focus on the factors that lead people either to seek medical assistance or to comply (or not to comply) with physicians' instructions. The assumption seems to be that patients play an active role before they get to doctors' offices and after they leave but that, while they are there, they are the passive puppets of doctors' orders. [12]

I believe that the relationship between doctor and patient can be characterized as a process of bargaining for control over the situation. The fact that one negotiator is in a weaker bargaining position than the other does not obviate the fact that a negotiation is taking place. Patients should be considered not passive role players but strategists who seek to overcome their limited roles to obtain the best possible outcomes.

The utility of viewing patients as strategists has been demonstrated in several insightful sociological studies. David Hayes-Bautista has described the medical encounter as a bargaining session in which patients try to influence the recommendations doctors make through such strategies as demanding or suggesting modifications in treatment regimens, disclosing new information, or asking leading questions. According to Hayes-Bautista, doctors respond to these patient strategies by overwhelming patients with expertise, threatening them with dire consequences if they do not comply with doctors' orders, explaining the rationale for the steps they have taken, or using "personal tactics." [13]

Julius Roth has described the hospital emergency room as the scene of negotiations for service. Staff, according to Roth's description try to control clients' behavior and protect physicians' time by keeping clients waiting and withholding information. Clients can take control of their own fate by being demanding, presenting their symptoms dramatically, relying on "connections," using their knowledge of emergency room operations, or taking advantage of lapses in the staff's attempts at information control. From his analysis of interaction in the emergency room Roth draws one main conclusion: The emergency room client is not at all a helpless pawn of the staff.[14]

In a discussion of people involved with alternative healing techniques, Meredith McGuire points out that many of these people use medical doctors in strategic ways. Subscribers to alternative healing techniques sometimes see medical doctors to rule out the possibility of a serious illness before going to an alternative healing practitioner for therapy. During the medical encounter such people often pretend to accept the medical model of reality lock, stock, and barrel when, in fact, they use doctors' services very selectively. McGuire describes these selective users of doctors' services as "contractors of their own health care."[15] But perhaps her most striking observation is that in this respect the users of alternative healing techniques were not terribly different from members of a control group—people not involved with alternative healing. All patients, it seems, use the medical encounter strategically.

I found that many people I interviewed, but especially the wives, acted as their own "fertility contractors." Like McGuire's users of alternative healing techniques and Roth's emergency room clients, they, too, acted strategically in an attempt to maximize their control over situations where they were defined as junior partners.[16]

One strategy for gaining control employed by many of those I interviewed involved attempts to become expert on the subject of infertility.[17] When I asked Lynn if the experience of infertility had changed her, she replied: "Well, I'm certainly wiser about the subject of fertility. I feel sometimes like I'm a walking dictionary." Fourteen wives and two husbands reported reading a lot about infertility. Many wives became absorbed with learning about the medical aspects of infertility, reading every related thing they could get their hands on and becoming lay experts. Karen contrasted her way of dealing with infertility to Brett's:

> You can't get rid of the pain; all you can do is try to. At least I try to have as much control of the situation as I can. One thing I do is read a lot. I go to the library and take out anything I can find on pregnancy and infertility. I've read every book in our library. I don't see it like grasping at straws because I'm not just trying any old thing that comes along. I just want to know more about what's happening to my body. My husband reads, but he doesn't read about infertility. He reads science fiction. I don't see him having that need to learn more about what's happening.

Other people relied on fertile and infertile friends as a source of information. For example, Sally said she talked to a lot of friends before mentioning to her gynecologist that she was having problems. Dan found one benefit of becoming involved with Resolve is that it gave him access to a storehouse of information: "It's good to be able to talk to people about what physician is doing what or who is sensitive or who is insensitive or what techniques are being used at what point in time."

In general, doctors are able to dominate medical encounters because they possess a monopoly on medical information.[18] Doctors' esoteric knowledge is, of course, not the only source of their power over patients, but it is a major source. Because patients depend on doctors to impart critical information, they often find it expedient to let doctors exert a high degree of control over the course of the medical encounter. Clearly, then, any steps patients take to expand their base of knowledge should give them a greater degree of control over the situation.

A number of wives used information about infertility as a tool to influence their gynecologists to accept their timetables for treatment.

Cathy's reading allowed her to devise a strategy to persuade her doctor to take her infertility seriously even though she and Chip had been trying for only seven months:

> I was very well read when we started. I think I just felt extremely confident about my knowledge on how to get pregnant and on recognizing when I was ovulating. After just a few months I was starting to wonder, and after about seven months I was convinced that there was something holding up the show. By seven months, I already had five temperature charts in my hand, and I walked into my doctor's office and said, "I'm not waiting twelve months to start."

Knowing that her doctor might not be willing to begin a workup after only four months of trying, Lynn lied to her doctor in an attempt to make sure he took her seriously: "First of all, I fibbed. I told him I had been trying six months instead of four months. But I didn't want to quibble and have him say, 'Oh, come back in a couple of months.' I was ready then, so I figured I'll cross my fingers and say six months."

Sally used her knowledge of the infertility workup creatively to speed the medical process along:

> Somebody had told me that, if you call your doctor and tell him that you're having problems, he's going to tell you that you have to wait a year and have three months of temperature charts. So I made up some temperature charts. I took my temperature for one month, and then I made up two more. And then I went to see him. So he took care of everything all at once and didn't say that I had to wait a year or anything.

Some wives made treatment suggestions to their doctors based on their reading. Liz began to suspect that she had tubal problems and insisted that her doctor perform a second hysterosalpingogram. Cathy asked her doctor to test her and Chip for a mycoplasma infection. In both of these cases, the wives' suspicions turned out to be justified.

Wives often sensed that their doctors felt threatened by their knowledge about infertility. Lynn saw her infertility expertise as a source of tension between herself and her doctor: "I think he thinks I was picking this up out of *Good Housekeeping* or something. I mean, I was going in there with *Journal of the American Medical Association* articles, going, 'Look, this study was done, and this and this and this.' So I was getting very frustrated at that point."

One strategy wives commonly used to exert more influence over the treatment process was to change doctors. Barbara called switching physicians a "big step in gaining some control." Wives unable or unwilling to persuade their physicians to modify the treatment regimen in accordance with their wishes often "voted with their feet." One frequently cited reason for switching was dissatisfaction with the slow progress of the treatment process. Mary switched to an infertility specialist because her gynecologist did not seem to accord the same significance to her problem as she did:

> I talked to my gynecologist about it, and he said, "Wait, relax. Sometimes it takes a year; sometimes it takes two years. If nothing happens in a year come back and see me." So we proceeded for another nine months, and then I went back and saw him. And he still said he didn't think there was anything wrong. He just said to continue onward, and if nothing happened we could go and have the sperm test, but he didn't get moving with the testing. That's when we switched to an infertility specialist.

As far as I can discern, no one in my sample switched from a gynecologist to an infertility specialist because of a referral. Wives left their gynecologists out of dissatisfaction, not because gynecologists had decided that the time had come to see a specialist. Rachel's gynecologist referred her to a specialist only after she "pushed": "After I pushed him, this gynecologist recommended a fertility specialist.

At that point, I decided it was probably time to take matters into my own hands, and I went and saw a different specialist." As this quotation illustrates, Rachel, like many other wives I talked with, saw switching doctors as a means of gaining more control over her own fate.

Switchers typically chose their own doctors carefully and prepared the ground well to assure they would be satisfied with their choices. Cathy called a number of gynecological practices before selecting her new doctor: "I called up specifically saying, 'Is this doctor interested in infertility, and is he up on the latest advancements in treating it?' And so he knew that was why I was coming to him. He didn't hesitate at all." According to Mike, he and Barbara did informal research among their friends before choosing a new physician: "Dr. McEwen was recommended by some friends. We talked to a lot of friends before we made any changes. You know, 'Who are you seeing? Are you happy with them?'" In addition, Barbara made sure that her new doctor was aware of the causes of her dissatisfaction with her previous physician: "I went to Dr. McEwen and explained to him just why I switched physicians. That was probably the best therapeutic session I had because then Dr. McEwen was aware of where I was coming from and just what problems I had with Dr. Robinson. And from then on I felt I had a special relationship with Dr. McEwen."

In these paragraphs I have been suggesting that it is more appropriate to view these infertility patients as active strategists rather than as passive recipients of health care. In some cases, couples had worked out for themselves quite elaborate game plans. Often, couples' plans combined medical and nonmedical solutions. Many couples viewed adoption as "an ace in the hole" that could be played when they became discouraged with their prospects for medical treatment. Debby turned to adoption when she began to feel impatient with the way things were going: "I had turned thirty right after I had the surgery, and I wasn't going to wait any longer. I went with the idea that now that I'm thirty, I better get going."

According to Barbara, she and Mike had developed a two-stage approach in their quest for a child:

> If life isn't going according to plan, it's time to make some new plans. That's when I made my New Year's resolution of, "If we don't have a biological child by December or it doesn't look like we're pregnant by December, then we'll look into adoption." So I figured, okay, if Plan A, which is having a biological child, doesn't work out, Plan B, having an adopted child, will be the next step.

While Barbara and Mike had decided to pursue adoption as their fall-back option if medical treatment failed, Karen and Brett decided to follow up on both options simultaneously. Karen explained:

> We're completing the paperwork to make the application for adoption now. The hormone regimen has been extremely difficult. It has kind of put me on a roller coaster. My moods go up and down, and my cycle's just all crazy with all these different hormones I'm on. And I don't know how long my body can really tolerate this craziness. On the other hand, I still want to give it the best shot we've got. The adoption would take a year to go through, so we're going to give the different medicines and stuff a year. At the end of that year, we will either have gotten pregnant through the medicines or we will have the adoption completed. So, one way or another, at the end of the year, we should have a child.

As one last example of the complexity of the infertility strategies developed by some couples, I quote at length from Cathy's description of what she and Chip were thinking as they entered an IVF program:

> Because we didn't expect it to work, we had this whole plan laid out. We were going to try IVF for as many times as we could

afford. Our insurance was going to dictate to us how many times we could attempt that, and—assuming that there would be probably two or three months between each attempt—we figured, "Okay, let's assume we're going to try that three times and that's going to take nine months to do. In the meantime, they'll have perfected this new sperm wash that they've come out with which is supposed to be very helpful when the motility is low. So, then we'll try that for a few months, and—after we've tried that for a few months—we'll make a decision as to whether we try AID. And, either after we've tried that or once we've decided not to try that, then we will start on a second adoption.

Given the use of the strategies I have been describing, it does not seem inappropriate to describe the couples I interviewed, but especially the wives, as "infertility contractors." While attempting to gain more control over their lives, they took on the responsibility of stage managing their treatment careers. They were not passive recipients of doctors' orders; rather they were independent contractors who worked hard to assure that doctors gave orders they found appropriate. Nor were they passive vis-à-vis their husbands. Contrary to what one might expect, wives typically exercised more influence than their husbands over the pace and direction of the treatment process.

It is important to remember that most wives in my sample were educated, middle-class women. Such women may be presumed more comfortable with the role of infertility contractor than workingclass or lower-class women might be. These wives' strategies would appeal to women who are relatively confident in their intellectual and communication skills. Employing these strategies requires faith in one's abilities both to understand technical written material and master technical jargon. Presumably, women with less education might find such strategies less natural.

Still, the role of infertility contractor did not come easily to everyone. Some wives found it difficult to move beyond the notion that a good patient was one who obeyed her doctor. Peg accepted this model of doctor-patient relations when she began her infertility workup:

> I don't know the exact year when things started to change. Now, more people are demanding more information about what's going on. But back then, you just trusted your doctor. If the doctor said you needed this, you said, "Oh, must be I need it." You know, you didn't question the doctor. He was the one that had all the knowledge, and you just didn't question it.

Over the course of the years when she was being treated for infertility, Liz came gradually to have more faith in herself and less in her doctors: "I have much less faith in them. I realize how many mistakes they make. Before I used to think they were quite perfect. I don't have the feeling that they really care." It is impossible to know whether the lessons some of these wives learned in the course of infertility treatment will carry over into other aspects of their lives. If these lessons do have any indirect long-term effects, then the experience of infertility may paradoxically give them a greater sense of control over at least some aspects of their everyday lives.

I have been making much of the fact that the infertile wives I talked to played an active role in trying to push their medical treatment in the way they wanted it to go. In general, they wanted it to go faster. Wives were often annoyed that their doctors did not seem to be taking them seriously enough, and they were often frustrated with the slow pace of progress.[19] The strategies I have been describing were, for the most part, deployed in an effort to move the treatment process along. It would not be completely appropriate, however, to describe wives' approach to infertility as "treatment-oriented." Rather, wives were "baby-oriented." Wives' strategies were directed, by and large, toward getting a baby as soon as possible. As long as the pursuit of treatment seemed to promise a baby in the foreseeable future, wives were treatment-oriented. But when treatment lost some of its promise, many became more focused on adoption. It may be useful to describe the orientation of infertile wives in terms of an "imperative for action."

Infertile women are sometimes portrayed as pressured by the medical profession into pursuing treatment. This is not what I observed among the wives I interviewed. Especially at the earlier stages of their treatment careers, *wives* worked to coax their *physicians* into a more active stance. As we see later in this chapter, however, doctors may have exerted some pressure on some wives to continue treatment when they might have been ready to call it quits. Doctors' actions may have, in some cases, acted to transmute wives' desires for babies into more specific desires to pursue treatment.

COMPASSION AND COMPETENCE

It seems clear that, far from accepting their doctors' actions and decisions on blind faith, these patients played an active role in evaluating their physicians. Patients had two standards against which they judged doctors: they expected doctors to be both competent and compassionate. They demanded of their doctors that they be experts in their field, but they also expected them to be sensitive to the emotional impact of infertility. They wanted their physicians to be humane and communicate a caring attitude through their demeanor. It was not always easy to find both qualities in the same person. For this reason, Kim stayed with her gynecologist even though she found him to be insensitive to the emotional needs of his infertile patients: "He is located in an Ob/Gyn clinic, so you're surrounded by your basic nineteen-year-olds and twelve-year-olds. I mean, really, everybody's pregnant. He even has this obnoxious statue on the checkout counter of a pregnant person that says, 'I should have danced all night.' Ughh! It's one of the worst places to be when you're in our shoes. On the other hand, he's a good doctor. So what do you do?"

Respondents often criticized gynecologists and urologists for not being knowledgeable about infertility. Dan complained about one of the several urologists he had visited:

I really felt like, in the field of infertility at any rate, he was incredibly naive. He didn't know what the hell he was doing. He might be a very good urologist, but he shouldn't have anything to do with infertility. He was guessing. It was like looking through a cookbook. "Look at this; we haven't tried this one. How about this?" And a couple times we suggested things to him, and he said, "Gee, I never thought of that. Why don't we try that one?" So we were being our own physicians.

Lynn had a similar story to tell about the first gynecologist she went to:

I truly believe he was trying to be an infertility specialist when in fact he's just an Ob/Gyn. And he's delivering babies and doing hysterectomies and everything else and just didn't have time. I mean, often I left feeling I knew more than him. And I was telling him things, and he was going, "Oh, really?" And I'm thinking, "Wait a minute, I'm paying you for this."[20]

Patients who had switched to infertility specialists were often more satisfied with their physicians' level of competence, but—in many cases—they still complained about lack of sensitivity. By and large, the couples in my sample felt their doctors focused on the organic aspects of infertility and paid little attention to infertility as a personal and emotional crisis.[21] Dan complained about what he saw as insensitivity on the part of most infertility specialists: "I think that, for the most part from what we've seen, there are more people who are insensitive and callous in the field than there are people who are sensitive and caring." Martha felt that the specialists she visited had a "narrow" outlook:

I felt positively about their expertise. I felt like they knew what they were doing. I never felt that they were fly-by-nighters or that they were just taking my money or anything like that. But, on the other hand, I think they were very narrow in their view. They're looking just at the physical aspect of conception, and I don't think they realize what a miracle it is, that there's more to life than just a sperm and an egg coming together.

Mary felt her doctor was not interested in her as a person: "I think, because he was into research, his primary concern was solving infertility problems, but I don't think he was really concerned about solving the patient's problem." Lee was disappointed that his doctor didn't seem to put much energy into the personal side of the doctor-patient relationship: "He's always in a hurry, and he doesn't even want to sit down and talk with you and explain things. He was very cold and very impersonal. I didn't care for him. He'd just come in and examine you and then just rush off and not really explain what he was doing. He leaves you in the dark and makes you wonder." Jim expressed his opinion of his urologist briefly: "Talking to my doctor was like talking to the siding on my house."

Patients, however, expressed considerable admiration and appreciation for doctors whom they saw as "sensitive." Sherry talked about the things her gynecologist did to make her patients feel more comfortable: "With my gynecologist, the towel that you cover yourself up with is sewed by somebody. It's a piece of fabric. You know, that kind of thing. The stirrups that you put your legs in are padded and covered and in color. Before they put the speculum in, they run it under warm water so that it's not a shock to the body." Sherry was grateful to have a doctor who treated her as much more than simply a patient:

> My doctor has been really fabulous. There was a point where I felt, if we ever had a child, I'd name it after her. I had very intense feelings toward her. She was really supportive. When we got the first bad news here from the urologist, I walked in to her office—it was lunch hour, and she was eating her lunch—and I cried with her. We were with her for over an hour, and she didn't charge us a penny.

When I asked Rachel why she liked her current doctor more than her first doctor, she replied: "Just more honest, I think. More willing to share with you the details of your case, your situation. More caring, a lot more caring. When I was in the hospital with the ectopic pregnancy, he must have spent hours with me. It really helped. You know, just different. You don't feel like you're a number; you feel like you're a person."

Hospitals were judged according to the same criteria used to judge physicians. Even when people saw hospital staff as competent, they were still critical of staff they saw as insensitive and of institutional arrangements that seemed indicative of insensitivity. When Jean went to the hospital for tubal surgery, she was very upset to find herself on the same floor with pregnant women:

> My hospital experience was not real good. When I had my surgery, they put all Ob/Gyn patients on the same floor. We got off the elevator on the floor, and right as soon as the elevator doors opened there was a sign to tell you how to get to the nursery. It was painted with balloons all over it. They usually separate OBs on one end of the floor and GYNs on the other. But they had an awful lot of babies born, and they ran out of rooms in the OB section. So they had babies down in the section where I was. And that was real hard to deal with, especially the night before my surgery. There was a baby in the room next door, and the baby cried all night. I was a nervous wreck. It was just real hard.

Jean also remembered vividly an insensitive remark made to her by a staff member:

> I think the worst thing was when a nurse's aide came in one day because I had to have tape over my incisions before I went into the shower. So she came in to tape me up, and she said, "Oh, did you have an operation to have no more babies?" First of all, it was none of her business, and second of all, if you're

going to ask stupid questions, check out who you're talking to first. And that was really hard.

But while they berated physicians and other hospital staff for their insensitivity, the people I spoke to usually exempted nurses from their criticisms. Nurses were seen as being more compassionate than doctors. Carol was appreciative of the nursing care she received: "The nurses were much better. In fact, I'm thinking of one who the doctor yelled at because she was holding my hand through some procedure—I can't remember which one. She said, 'Oh, she really needs me right here.' That was really nice." Liz also remembered her nurses fondly: "They really cared. They remembered your name, and where you lived. Maybe because most of them were mothers, they could understand how much I wanted to get pregnant. Maybe it's because we're the same sex, and we could just you know . . . . And they had more time; they weren't rushed. It wasn't the same five minutes in, give you the shot, then take off again." And Rick remembered one nurse in particular: "There was one nurse there that was so good. She was just so super, I'll never even forget her name. Her name was Marie. She was just very patient, very caring. She was the one who got me out walking around."

Thus, although some people I spoke with were more satisfied about their interactions with health care personnel than were others, there was a remarkable degree of consensus about the criteria upon which health care personnel were to be judged. Both infertile wives and husbands looked for competence and sensitivity from physicians, nurses, and other staff.

THE EXPERIENCE OF TREATMENT

Patients' experiences of treatment are, of course, affected by many other factors than the quality of their interactions with medical staff. Regardless of how they felt about their doctors and nurses, few—if any—people I interviewed remembered infertility treatment as pleasant. Some unpleasant treatment experiences people recalled might possibly have been prevented by more sensitive staff or by better-thought-out institutional arrangements, but some seemed intrinsic to the medical treatment of infertility. Some wives I spoke with complained that some diagnostic tests were painful. Carol complained about her hysterosalpingogram: "After a while, you felt like you were a whiner and a complainer, but I know that hurt. That wasn't my imagination; that hurt! It's not like just having a sperm count or something. There are very few things that they can do to a women that don't hurt."

Both husbands and wives found many of the tests they had to undergo embarrassing and humiliating. Jim recalled how he felt when he had to collect a semen sample in his doctor's office: "Well, I'll be frank about this. Jerking off for a test is terrible. I thought being on a video camera on a closed circuit TV doing a sales pitch or learning a sales routine was embarrassing. No, that session in the can beat it by a long shot." Chip's experience with semen analysis was "terrible":

> I mean, that was terrible. You walked into a waiting room—
> it was an office in the hospital—and there were probably, you
> know, a few couches, tables, and so on around, and one recep-
> tionist. And you walked in, and she takes your name and hands
> you a bottle. And she says, "Go have a seat." So you go have a
> seat hanging on to your little cup, along with all these other
> people sitting in there with their little cups, all trying not to
> look at each other and trying not to feel embarrassed. Cathy was
> with me, and this friend of ours who was in Boston was with us.
> So we're sitting there waiting, and somebody comes in from the
> bathroom down the hall with the key. Well, then that's when
> the next person gets up and goes. So you see somebody come
> back with one of these keys, like gas station keys, a big board
> like this with a key on the end. And then, when he comes back,
> it's your turn, so you grab the key and go. You take your key and
> your cup, and you go down the hall to this bathroom which at
> night must double as a janitor's room. I mean it was huge, and

all it had in it was a toilet and a sink and an open closet with brooms and dust mops and all that stuff in it. It was just pathetic, absolutely pathetic.

But what made it even worse was that, once you have done your business and you come back with your cup in your hand, that's where you sit. You sit and wait, and you've got this thing in your hand. I mean, what do you do with it? You're sitting there with it, and while, yes, all you guys are in the same situation, it's still kind of uncomfortable. And besides that there were the wives and so on that are with these people. And you sit there with this cup in your hand waiting because when the doctor finally calls you, you walk in with it. I mean, I just was totally turned off by that whole operation down there. I just couldn't believe it was that bad. It was just unbelievable. Their style of doing it was terrible. The doctor was nice, a very friendly guy, a very nice guy. But that way of doing things was just terrible.

Wives who had undergone artificial insemination sometimes found that experience especially unsavory. Martha described her encounter with AID:

I was always very nervous whenever I went up there. The whole situation was really kind of sleazy. He used fresh semen so, when you got there, he would run out and get whoever it was to give him the sample, and then I would have to pay him in cash. So after you had this thing done, you have to slip him this twenty-five dollars. It was just . . . . [sigh] "You went into this sterile examining room, and it was on one of those OB tables with the stirrups and everything and this florescent light glaring down on you. And then after he'd do it, he would say, "Well, good luck," and he'd walk out. You're left laying on this table, and you can't move for twenty minutes.

Lois and Stuart were especially eloquent in describing their treatment experiences. Stuart said he found the entire treatment process embarrassing:

> As far as the testing and things like that go in infertility, it annoyed me a lot. I guess I felt like you're exposing your most private and personal thoughts to complete strangers. And it almost gets to the point where you want to say, "The hell with it all," because you don't want to even have to talk about the stuff or discuss it with somebody.

Lois was especially bothered by the postcoital test:

> I think the hardest was when I knew I had to go through that postcoital thing. I almost felt like the cameras were on me or something. I know no one else was around, but it was like . . . oh, my God! I go walking out and stare at the girls behind the counter. They know why I'm there, and the doctor knows, and even my mother's at home thinking. . . . Well, I'm sure she wasn't, but I felt so self-conscious.

At one point in our interview, Lois talked about her sense that she had lost her dignity:

> By the time I ended up in the hospital—this was after I had probably five or six tests—I'd swear I'd probably pull down my pants for anyone that walked by because I'd lost all of my dignity. I'm a very modest person, but I began to feel like I was a car being worked on. You know, all these throngs of people were all over you. I know that postcoital test was very embarrassing.

Peg spoke for many when she described infertility treatment as dehumanizing: "It really wears at you after a while. You have so many doctors poking and prodding you and telling you this and telling you that. You become a specimen almost, rather than a human being. It gets to you."

A number of the people I interviewed complained about the long duration of the infertility treatment process. Rachel spoke of her feeling that, although she and Tom had been in treatment for two years, they didn't seem to be getting anywhere: "It had been two years, and we still hadn't done anything to treat it. I guess that's what really made me upset. We had been going at this for two years, and we had been doing all sorts of testing. But we never really did anything to correct the problem." Chip expressed annoyance with the slow progress he and Cathy experienced in their attempt to have a child: "It would seem that the process could be sped up some. Let's get through this testing. I'm not saying doing it one after another and not leave any time, but, let's get through this process, let's find out what's going on."

People also voiced frustration at the sense of uncertainty that pervaded the infertility treatment process. Karen said:

> We're just so used to taking a drug and having it get all better. But this isn't that kind of thing. You've got to juggle the medicines and whatever until you find the right combination. It seems real hard to accept that, with all the medical technology they've got, they don't have an easy pat way of saying, "Yes, this is exactly your problem and this is exactly how we treat it." They don't have that.

Rachel raised the issue of lost control as she expressed her frustration that medical technology cannot provide her with the certainty she wants so badly: "It's just incredibly frustrating. I think that the most frustrating thing for me was the loss of control. There was nothing that I could do. You go through all these procedures, all these tests, all these pills, but there is nothing that is going to guarantee that you are going to get pregnant."

The meaning of the absence of signs of physiological malfunction appears quite different for infertility than for most cases of illness. In illness, a doctor's inability to find a serious physical impairment is usually (though not always) regarded as good news. But, in infertility, not having a diagnosable physical impairment is no guarantee that a couple will achieve pregnancy, as a quotation from Richard illustrates:

> The doctor, after all the surgeries, more or less said, "Hey, you're ready to go. There's no reason that you shouldn't have a kid." Which is sometimes worse than having someone say that you're not ever going to have a kid. And we don't know why it's not happening. So we liken it to a constant grieving process unlike where someone dies and you grieve for x number of weeks or months, and you bury them.

Another feature of the experience of infertility worth noting— briefly mentioned in Chapter 3—is its engulfing nature. In Chapter 2, I drew attention to the analogy between infertility and chronic illness. As with chronic illness, the infertility treatment regimen can easily overshadow other aspects of patients' lives.[22] The demands of the treatment regimen remain constantly in the background of everyday life and often intrude into the foreground. Cindy said that infertility was constantly on her mind: "You had to be at the doctor all the time or on the phone or something, you know. And then we had to not have sex so often and then have it and . . . . I don't know; I can't remember it all anymore. But it was on my mind all the time then." Kim felt she never had a day off: "It seemed that, whenever it was my time to ovulate, it was a weekend or holiday. I'm not kidding you. Memorial Day weekend, Fourth of July, I hit them all. I'd meet Dr. Singh in the parking lot of his office, and we'd walk in together." And Jean described infertility as a life-style:

> Infertility gets to be a life-style after a while. You start your day with a thermometer in your mouth. You always know what day of your cycle it is. You always know when your period is

coming or should be coming, and you hope it won't. When I was on clomiphene citrate, it was always Wednesday five to nine. That's when I had to take my clomiphene citrate, and if I was going away I had to be sure I had it with me. And I had to be at the doctor on this and this and this day. It becomes like an obsession after a while.

Earlier, I drew attention to the paradox of control that confronts infertile couples, especially wives. A desire to regain a sense of control over their lives leads them to enter into situations in which their sense of control is threatened still further. This section has illustrated some ways in which infertility treatment can threaten patients' sense of control. To attain a sense of normalcy, the infertile pursue a course of action that often leads to pain and humiliation, that dwarfs other aspects of their lives, that is long term in its duration and uncertain in its outcome.

STOPPING

Hearing infertile people describe the experience of infertility treatment in such vivid terms might lead one to ask why people would subject themselves to such conditions. After all, infertility is not life-threatening. Unlike cancer patients, for example, whose only alternative to a painful treatment regimen may be death, the infertile do have a genuine choice. They could refuse to continue treatment. Thus, it is striking that the infertile are, as a rule, quite committed to pursuing treatment. According to journalist Marsha Stamell, infertility patients are surpassed only by cancer patients in their willingness to subject themselves to costly, painful, and sometimes hopeless medical procedures.[23]

No couple in my sample have reconciled themselves to childfree living.[24] Even Kate and Roger, who had not pursued treatment by the time of the interview had decided that it was time for Kate, at age forty-one, to begin an infertility workup. Once they had begun treatment, people found it very difficult to stop. Other wives also testify to the difficulty they had in calling an end to treatment. Debby recalled: "After the laparoscopy, I called my husband and said, 'I will never do anything like this again.' And two weeks later, I went in and had the surgery. I guess I kept feeling like I wanted to try." Martha said she could just not bring herself to give up on the idea of becoming pregnant: "Several times I've said, 'This is it.' You know, when you come out of surgery and you're throwing up all over the place and you're sicker than a dog, you say, 'I'm not going to go through this again. This is ridiculous.' Then things happen, and you just. . . . I just can't believe that I physically can't get pregnant. I just can't believe that."

Husbands were generally more willing than wives to stop treatment, even if they themselves had reproductive impairments. Jean spoke of the difference between her point of view and Rick's: "Especially after our adopted son came, it was much easier for Rick. He could have cared less at that point as far as pursuing with doctors and that. I think it was hard for him to understand why I still had a need to be pregnant. I think it's still hard for him to understand."

One factor that may make stopping difficult is related to the uncertain, open-ended nature of infertility. The same factors that make it possible for infertile couples to hope realistically for a child can make it quite hard for the members of an infertile couple to concede their condition may be permanent. The fact that there is almost always another step that can be taken strengthens the imperative for action and makes infertility harder to accept.[25] Richard revealed how the open-ended nature of infertility can pose problems: "I think there's a sense of ambiguity when so many things can happen, when you still hold out hope it may happen one day. I've talked with other people who seem in a sense almost relieved because they've been told they'll never have children. They just start to adopt, and they think about other things, and they don't worry about that." Sherry and Dan had given up on treatment until they learned about a new option that had become available: "We stopped. I though we were all finished last year until I had done more research. Actually I wasn't even looking.

It was just something I read in the Resolve newsletter. We both thought we were done."

The imperative for action may be strengthened for these couples by the feeling that time is running out. The infertile couples I spoke to conveyed a strong awareness of the pressure of time. They were acutely aware that the possibility of becoming parents would not remain open forever. They were quite anxious to achieve parenthood before they passed the not very clearly defined ages beyond which biological parenthood would be unattainable. As Craig put it: "The fact that we are becoming older, that time was biologically running out for us, led to the desire to seek whatever types of medical attention that were available."

Couples' decisions to halt treatment did not usually mean that they had given up the pursuit of parenthood. Stopping medical treatments did not mean giving up on parenthood, only on biological parenthood. Often the decision to call a halt to treatment was accompanied by developing or renewing a commitment to actively pursue adoption. The ways in which people talked about the reasons they stopped treatment show clearly that they saw stopping as consistent with the imperative for action. Karen outlined the reasons she and Brett decided not to pursue IVF:

> My husband went to the workshops on finances, and one of the ones that he attended was dealing with the IVF stuff. He came out and said, "I don't think that's going to be an option for us." You are looking at five thousand dollars a try and no guarantee of any results, and he says if we had five thousand dollars, we'd put it toward adoption and at least be guaranteed of getting a child.

Kim related her reasons for deciding to pursue adoption: "It became clear to me that, being the impatient person that I am, I had it with this medical junk. It wasn't working. I was doctor hopping, we were city hopping, and we were getting nowhere. And I didn't need to be pregnant. That became real clear to me. I just wanted to bag it. I wanted a child ASAP."

Couples called a halt to treatment when they ran out of options or when they "burned out." According to Lois, she and Stuart had no choice but to stop trying:

> The only other thing we could try was IVF. And most medical insurance doesn't cover the cost of that. We read up on that a lot. We even called the research center at the university and talked with them about it. They said that there's a very low probability of getting pregnant. And sometimes it takes five or six times before it works. I think it was like five thousand or ten thousand dollars every time you did it. It's very uncomfortable for the woman. She would have to be out of work for a period of time every time they did it. So as far as I'm concerned, there were no more options.

It should be noted here that "running out of options" is a matter of definition rather than an objectively defined medical state. From a medical point of view, Lois and Stuart still had options. They could have pursued IVF, but—when they thought about what that would mean for their finances, their emotional well-being, their style of life, and the possibility of adopting—they decided it was not a viable option for them. Being without options is not an objective state that couples reach; rather, couples must *decide* that they have run out of options.

Jean said she quit because she was sick of treatment: "I was just sick of clomiphene citrate. I was sick of going to the doctors all of the time. I was sick of the bills. I was really sick of it. I just had to get over it, so we just finally gave ourselves a deadline and said that we are going to get to this point and that's going to be it. And we stuck to it." According to Peter, he and Kim just burned out: "We burned out. Kim is running to various doctors here, and we're going to this place and that place, and the end result of all of that time and energy and money was—nothing. So we just burned out and had to stop the medical stuff."

Although running out of options and burning out appear to be different reasons for ending treatment, in reality they seem to me to be two different idioms couples employ to make the same basic point; they are two different ways to express the idea that couples stop treatment when they decide that they would do better to channel their energies in other directions. It is not surprising that, without objective criteria to rely upon, couples find it difficult to close the door on the pursuit of medical treatment.

In some cases, physicians may act in ways that make it more difficult to halt treatment.[26] Dee described what she saw as pressure from her physician to keep pursuing treatment: "I said, 'No more. I'm not doing this anymore.' So I stopped, and I didn't go to the doctor for a while. Then I had to go because I had an infection. He wanted to talk to me about infertility. I told him I couldn't at this time. I came to talk to him about the infection and that was all." The pressure to pursue treatment is not always limited to the realm of doctor-patient interaction. Judith Lasker and Susan Borg report seeing a sign in the waiting room of an IVF clinic that read, "You never fail until you stop trying."[27]

INFERTILITY AS LIMINALITY

We have seen that the uncertainty of infertility made it difficult for infertile couples to opt out of treatment. I believe that uncertainty is a critical feature of the contemporary experience of infertility.

The British medical sociologist Michael Bury has used the term "biographical disruption" to describe the experience of the chronically ill, who discover in midcourse that their lives are not likely to conform to their life plans.[28] Biographical disruption also seems appropriate for describing the experience of the infertile. Infertility presents itself not simply as a failure of the reproductive system but as a radical threat to life plans that had seemed to be moving according to schedule.

The experience of infertility can be characterized as an experience of "status blockage": the infertile are prevented from achieving a status—that of parenthood—they find desirable, if not essential.[29] The infertile are thereby deterred from fulfilling their own expectations of what it means to be an adult in American society. But, it is essential to note that the infertile do not see the status of parenthood as something removed from their grasp once and for all. Because of the uncertainty of the infertility trajectory, the majority of the infertile have good reason to harbor the hope that they may still achieve the status of parenthood. They do not necessarily see themselves as permanently childless; rather, they see themselves as *not yet pregnant*.

Sociologists Ralph Matthews and Anne Martin Matthews describe the experience of infertility as a transition to the status of non-parenthood, but it would be more accurate to describe it as a transition to "statuslessness." To use a term popularized by social anthropologist Victor Turner, the infertile are characterized by *liminality*. They are "betwixt and between"—no longer children but unable to fully play the role of adult as Americans perceive it. In his study of the transition to the identity of adoptive parenthood, Kerry Daly describes this process as one that moves by fits and starts, characterized by "creative bumbling."[30] Given the uncertainty of the infertility trajectory, parenthood for the infertile is a status that can be neither achieved nor abandoned. Barbara clearly voiced this sense of liminality: "I didn't fit into any category. I still don't fit into any category right now." Martha, too, characterized herself as being in limbo: "I would say, for the past two years, I've sort of been putting things on hold. That's been a lot of my problem. I think my life has always been moving along, and now things are sort of [sigh]. . . . I'm not going anywhere."

To summarize, the infertile wives in my sample both wanted and expected to achieve motherhood, which they saw as integral to what it means to be a woman. When it became evident that it would be difficult or impossible to achieve this desired status, they were shocked. But, because they saw infertility as "curable" and their infertile status as transitional they focused their attention not on the need to adjust to their status but on its intolerability.

The uncertainty associated with infertility today means it is difficult to see the goal of biological parenthood as unachievable, one that ought to be rejected. Thus, it is not surprising that infertile couples, especially infertile wives, seem so willing to subject themselves to a demanding and often dehumanizing treatment regimen.

FIVE

TOGETHER APART
Issues of Communication and Intimacy

Over the past twenty years or so, a new ideal for marriage has become popular in the United States.[1] This new "marriage norm" holds that the good marriage is one in which husband and wife can communicate openly and freely on all subjects. The nineteenth-century doctrine of the two spheres is slowly giving way to the idea that husbands and wives are mutually responsible for their own and their spouses' continued growth and development.

COMMUNICATION AND INTIMACY
IN AMERICAN MARRIAGE

This new ideal for marriage flies in the face of long-standing expectations for men to be rational and unemotional and for women to be sensitive and empathetic. Wives have long been regarded as responsible for overseeing the emotional health of their marriages, and some evidence shows that wives tend to live up to these expectations. Research has shown that wives are more disposed than husbands to disclose "negative" emotions. Wives are more likely than their husbands to monitor and orchestrate intimacy. They have been found more sensitive than their husbands to what is going on in their marriages and more likely to bring important issues in a relationship up for discussion. In marital discussions, wives tend to rely more on emotional appeals while husbands make an effort to stay "calm and reasonable."[2]

Sociologist Francesca Cancian has argued that the new ideal of the "communicative marriage" exalts traditionally feminine styles of intimacy and denigrates masculine styles through its equation of intimacy with talking. In American society, women tend to express intimacy in close relationships by sharing feelings and offering support; the masculine style of intimacy, on the other hand, emphasizes shared activity. For women, closeness tends to mean sharing one's most private feelings and empathizing with others when they express their feelings. For men, closeness more often involves doing things for or with another person. Much literature shows that wives *are* more inclined toward expressiveness and self-disclosure than husbands. The new norms for marriage make what Cancian calls a "feminine style of love" into the ideal for both wives and husbands. Thus, the ideal of the "communicative marriage" makes it almost inevitable that men will be found wanting.[3]

One major dilemma of American marriage is that wives and husbands must try to please one another by acting in ways that neither accord with their socialization nor appeal to their sense of comfort. The new expectations for marriage have the potential to exacerbate this tension within American society. Tension produced by differences in wives' and husbands' needs for communication and intimacy is endemic in middle-class American families.[4] By accepting the ideal of the communicative marriage wives may raise expectations for their husbands' behavior; as a result, they may be less satisfied than before with the quality of intimacy in their marriages.

The new expectations for communicative marriage give rise to what sociologist and clinical psychologist Lilian Rubin calls the "approach-avoidance" script of American marriages in which wives complain that their husbands will not "talk" to them while husbands wonder what their wives want them to talk about. American wives and husbands, Rubin says, are "intimate strangers." They share the same house and the same bed, but—in terms of experience—they are worlds apart. The experiences of wives and husbands are so different that sociologist Jessie Bernard asserts that within every marriage there are two marriages: his and hers.[5] American marriage is an institutionalized struggle in which two people who have learned to approach the world in very different ways must strive to discover what they can share.

We have seen in Chapter 3 that the effects of infertility on identity differ dramatically for wives and husbands. I now examine the *shared* experience of infertility. What happens when two people, each affected differently by infertility, interact intimately with one another? In this chapter, I look at the ways the infertile wives and husbands I interviewed experienced their marital relationships, and I study the effects they felt infertility had upon their marriages.

INFERTILITY AS *HER* PROBLEM

As we saw in Chapter 3 only a few husbands spoke in terms that would lead us to believe they experienced infertility as evidence of their failure as men. When the husbands I interviewed did speak of infertility as a failure, they usually referred not to the role of "man" or "father" but rather "provider" or "protector." Dave, whose low sperm count made it extremely unlikely that he would ever father a child, recounted: "I still think that it's somewhat within my power to do something that could help Martha. And I'm frustrated that I can't. I'm really frustrated that I can't solve Martha's problems or contribute to the solution of them for her." Roger said: "I can usually make things better. If my daughter gets hurt, I can make her feel better. I can give her medicine. I can take her to the doctor. But here, I lost complete control."

Many husbands were upset not so much by the experience of infertility itself as by its effects on their wives and their relationships with their wives. Dave said: "I love Martha dearly and desperately, and as long as she's less than happy I'll never be really happy. I think that her lack of happiness is the main stumbling block in my life. Otherwise, my life is quite satisfactory." Tony contrasted his response to infertility to his wife Sally's response:

> I think she reacted a lot stronger in terms of her body not working, and it being her responsibility and not being a mother. I reacted and got angry more at the inconvenience and the unfairness of it. She took it more to heart and personally. I feel like I probably dealt more with her response. I probably got more frustrated by her response than by the whole thing just as myself.

Barbara described Mike's attitude toward infertility: "He was concerned but more concerned with my mental health than with actually having a child." Thus, both husbands and wives seemed to identify infertility as mainly the wife's problem. While wives seemed most concerned with the way infertility was affecting them, husbands were often more concerned with the way it was affecting their wives and their relationships with their wives.

My quantitative research with a clinic-based sample of 449 infertile couples supports the idea that husbands tend to respond to infertility indirectly through their wives rather than directly.[6] The strongest predictor of life satisfaction for both men and women in this sample was partner's life satisfaction. The number of different life spheres about which people reported worrying was also significantly related to life satisfaction for both men and women. Women's life satisfaction, however, was generally associated with a number of other variables not significantly related to men's life satisfaction—for instance, sexual satisfaction, whether the husband had a documented reproductive impairment, and how long the couple had been trying to conceive. In other words, it takes a fairly complex model to account for variations in life satisfaction among infertile women, but variations in life satisfaction among infertile men can be accounted for by a simpler model in which the main explanatory variable is partner's life satisfaction. I interpret these data as supporting the hypothesis that wives' responses to infertility are more direct while husbands' responses are mediated by their wives' responses.[7]

Even in situations where there was an obvious male reproductive impairment, the wife still tended to view the situation as her problem. Jim, who had a low sperm count and poor motility, described Mary's response to infertility:

> She assumed we would have a couple of kids, at least, and just do the storybook type of thing. And, when that didn't happen, she felt less of a woman because she couldn't have kids. She felt unworthy of my love because she couldn't provide me with any kids. So it didn't matter at all that I couldn't provide her. She seemingly overlooked that fact completely. She got into a situation where she really lacked self-confidence and needed a lot of support. She was really bummed.

The wives I spoke with tended to evaluate their husbands in terms of their support. For example, Martha complained that Dave had not been supportive enough: "You know, he's not overly supportive. When we were looking into adoption, he wasn't overly enthusiastic or supportive or saying, 'Did you write to so and so?' or 'Let's call so and so,' or 'Let's look into this agency,' or 'Let's begin the paperwork.' He didn't encourage in that way." Robin, on the other hand, saw Lee as being quite supportive: "He spent all his energy and all his time trying to make me feel better. He never spent a lot of time dwelling on his feelings. It was always how he could make me feel better." Later in the interview, Robin added: "I thought he was supportive. If he sat down and cried, I would have felt, 'Now I don't have anybody to turn to.' I needed somebody to be strong."

It is interesting to note that, while wives often spoke about their husbands as supportive and sometimes complained their husbands were not supportive enough, the term "supportive" was *never* used by a husband to describe a wife. An ideal husband was seen as one who would support his wife in *her* time of adversity. It is also interesting to note that the sense that the ideal husband is supportive was not limited to the wives who had a diagnosed reproductive impairment. Robin, who we have just heard describing Lee as supportive, had no diagnosed reproductive impairment; Lee, however, had a motility problem.

In all four cases where the husband, not the wife, had a diagnosed reproductive impairment, the wives harbored the suspicion that their bodies also must be working imperfectly. Sociologist Charlene Miall, describing situations where wives accept the stigma for their husbands' infertility, has designated them as instances of "courtesy stigma."[8] My data also show wives willingly taking responsibility for infertility when their husbands have physiological problems, but I don't think that the term "courtesy stigma" captures the reality these women experienced. They did not describe themselves as accepting responsibility for their husbands' infertility; rather, they still thought of themselves as *being infertile*.

TENSION IN RELATIONSHIPS

Considering the vast differences that exist between the ways in which wives and husbands experience infertility, it should come as no surprise that a number of the people I interviewed characterize relationships with their spouses as tense and frustrated. In eighteen of the twenty-two couples I spoke with, wives and husbands agreed that infertility had led to increased tension. In only one case did husband and wife agree that the experience of infertility had not resulted in increased tension.

A number of wives, including six of the ten wives whose husbands had diagnosed reproductive impairments, were distressed by the fact that their husbands were unwilling to participate in decisions as equal partners and that they didn't seem very affected by the experience of infertility. Some wives expressed annoyance that their husbands seemed relatively untouched by something the women saw as ruining their lives. Barbara described her anger at her husband Mike: "I would get really ticked off. I would say, 'How could you not let this affect you? It's affecting my whole life, and it just seems to be water off your back.'" Karen experienced Brett's lack of involvement with infertility as a sort of desertion. She expressed her sense of loneliness poignantly: "Sometimes I feel like I'm trying to get pregnant all by myself."

While wives were often frustrated because their husbands were less affected than they were by the problem of infertility, some husbands thought their wives were overreacting. Tom described himself as having had this attitude on occasion: "There were definitely times when I felt Rachel was too incensed. She was too involved. She was allowing it to rule too much of her life." Jeff got annoyed when he thought Teri was making their situation seem worse than it actually was:

A good friend of mine from high school and his wife were over last month, and they said, "When are you guys going to have children?" And my wife blurted out, "We can't have children!" And I just looked at her and said, "Now that's not true, you know that. That's silly." And then I explained to them that we've been trying and we haven't been successful. I wish she wouldn't couch it in those terms because we haven't had any tests that show that.

Many wives complained that their husbands seemed unwilling to really involve themselves in talking about infertility. When I asked Rachel if she and Tom talked about infertility much, she answered:

Sometimes, but he didn't really like to talk about it either. I guess he thought I was being obsessed with it. We talked more about what we were going to do than about how we felt. I guess that's the best way to put it. He just thought I was totally focused on it, which I was. But that was the only way I could deal with it. You know, it wasn't the most important thing in his life, and it was the most important thing in mine.

111

But, while wives wished for more communication, some husbands didn't know what there was to say. As we saw earlier, Martha did not think Dave was "encouraging" enough. But Dave thought he and Martha communicated "pretty well":

> *Interviewer:* Do you talk much about infertility, the two of you?
> *Dave:* A fair amount. We communicate pretty well, I think.
> *Interviewer:* Is it something that comes up once a week, once a month, everyday, once every couple of months?
> *Dave:* I'd say once a month. How much can you talk about something that there are no answers to?

Paul said he was tired of hearing Dee complain all the time: "She knows that I don't want to hear about it because she's thirty-three and she shouldn't be pissed off about something she can't help. That's the way I look at it. If it's something that her body can't do, it's something her body can't do, and she's just going to have to get used to it."

Thus, wives were often upset because their husbands were unwilling to talk to them about infertility, but husbands were often annoyed by their wives' insistence on talking when talking would make no practical difference. This clash of wives' and husbands' intimacy styles sometimes led to arguments among the infertile couples I interviewed. Karen was particularly adept at describing the nuances of her relationship with Brett:

> We've always had a communication difference in that I tend to communicate on an emotional level and he tends to communicate on a very practical level. It makes a good marriage because we have both ends of the spectrum covered. But when we want to talk about things, we have to work quite hard at it because I'm affected more emotionally by the infertility and he's affected more practically. For him, it's just not convenient. It's not convenient to have scheduled sex; it's not convenient to have to pay out all the money for the medicines. For him, it's more

the practical things and the fact that our plans for the future haven't worked out. And, in some instances, when we're trying to talk about things—you know, if the sex routine is getting us down or whatever—we have to work harder to communicate because we're affected at different levels.

Cathy recalled some of the "shock tactics" she used to try to encourage Chip to be more involved: "I remember saying, 'I'm not even sure that maybe this is the way it's meant to be because we just simply can't communicate. If we can't communicate on this, how are we going to communicate when we do have kids?' I kind of used that as an argument." Chip remembered Cathy's angry accusations vividly: "She'd get very upset with me. 'You don't seem to care, you don't seem to take an interest in this. How come you don't read the newsletters from Resolve? You didn't go to the Resolve meeting with me. Don't you care about this whole thing?'" Some couples did not argue so much; instead, they retreated from one another. According to Rachel, she and Tom pulled away from each other: "We'd argue, I guess, but not a lot. It would just pull us apart. We each sort of went our own separate way. That's the best way to describe it, I think. We got very, very separate."

In a few cases, the communication difficulties I am describing led to situations where husband and wife did not know where each other stood on a particular issue. When asked if he and his wife have considered adoption, Dave answered: "I'm all for it, but she thinks that I have problems with adopting children of other races, and I don't think I do."

Conflict over communication and intimacy is obviously not unique to infertile couples. As we have seen, contention over communication and intimacy is endemic in American marriages. Infertility is just one stage on which the American couple's intimacy approach-avoidance script is acted out. The tension I have just been describing regarding communication about infertility is simply a special case of wives' general tendency to reach out for greater communication and emotional support and husbands' general tendency to resist.

113

"IT BROUGHT US CLOSER TOGETHER"

Because differences in the way marital partners respond to infertility clearly lead to frequent tensions and difficult communication, we might reasonably expect the vast majority of infertile couples to report that their marriages are extremely unhappy. Although the wives and husbands I interviewed expressed feelings of frustration and concern over their communication problems, these marriages, however, were not on the verge of breaking up. In fact, half the individuals (twelve wives and twelve husbands) in the sample felt that infertility had brought them closer together. In nine of the couples I spoke to, husbands and wives agreed that infertility had brought them closer together. In four couples, however, both spouses thought they had become more distant from each other than before. One couple felt infertility had not affected their relationship, and eight couples sent "mixed signals."[9]

The fact that half of the people I interviewed said that infertility brought them closer together is made more impressive by the fact that these couples were not *prompted* to either affirm or deny that their relationships had been strengthened. The question to which they responded was not, Has infertility strengthened or weakened your relationship? Rather, they volunteered this interpretation in response to the open-ended question, How do you think infertility has affected your relationship?

Most writers who have based their opinions on impressions gleaned from counseling infertile couples have asserted that infertility poses a threat to marriage.[10] But results from the few research studies in which infertile couples have been systematically compared to fertile couples do not bear this out. To the contrary, such studies have found that infertility is related to improved marital communication and higher levels of marital satisfaction.[11]

How is it possible, given the differences in the ways wives and husbands experience infertility, for infertility to improve marital relationships? Perhaps a better understanding of the effects of infertility on marital intimacy can come from a closer look at the themes that emerge from my interviews with couples who saw infertility as having had a salutary effect on their marital relationships.

A number of the people who said that infertility had brought them closer together stressed the idea that infertility was a major life crisis and that they were forced to pull together to "weather the storm." Jean and Rick are typical of these people. According to Jean, "It brought us closer together. It was like a major life crisis that just didn't quit. It just went on and on and on. We felt a lot of the time like it was just going to be us against the world. Everything was facing us, and it was just the two of us that had to dig our way out." Richard said he felt that he and Debby had been tested: "I think my marriage has been solidified and that I know how much I want it to work. I know that it isn't all roses like it was for a long time. I feel like we've gone through a test, and I think in a lot of ways we've been tested more than some people have." And Debby agreed, "In the long run it's really made us stronger. It's forced us to deal with issues that a lot of other people haven't dealt with."

Confronting a crisis together, then, can be a force that binds marital partners together. In a study of parents of children with cancer, a team of psychologists also found that marital partners report that a crisis had improved the quality of their marital relationships.[12] Any crisis could produce this same effect, but infertility may be especially conducive to interpretations defining it as a shared crisis. We have seen in Chapter 2 that infertility differs from many other health problems precisely because it is generally seen as a problem for a couple rather than an individual. Therefore, couples confronting infertility may be even more likely to see themselves facing a shared problem than might couples confronting other kinds of crises.

"Pulling together" was a theme commonly sounded by the couples I spoke to. People who said that infertility had strengthened their marriage often described the desire to have a child as a common goal toward which they could strive together. As Liz put it: "I think it made us closer because we had a common problem sort of situation there. We were trying to achieve the goal of having a child. For one reason or another we couldn't, and we were trying together to solve the problem. So, in order to solve it, we had to pull together." Lynn was very explicit in describing one way in which she and Jack had to pull together:

> He gave me the shots of Perganol. He was taught to give me the intramuscular injections. I think that really gave us a sense of pulling together on it because I was not afraid to have him give me a shot and he was not afraid to give me a shot. If anything good can come of it, it was kind of a confidence builder to both of us that we could count on each other for that sort of thing.

"Talking a lot" is another theme mentioned frequently by the couples who say infertility strengthened their marriage. Carol said that sharing a common problem forced her and Bill to communicate: "More than most couples I know probably we have to depend on each other and our relationship to make our marriage work. We are both very aware of that, I think. So we do talk a lot." One study that compared involuntarily childless couples to a matched sample of couples with children found that the involuntarily childless couples had a higher degree of rapport than the couples with children.[13] This finding might stem from the fact that facing the crisis of infertility together led to better communication: better communication may, in turn, have led to greater rapport. In my sample also, increased communication seems associated with an increased sense of empathy. Teri said that infertility had put Jeff more in touch with her feelings:

> We're closer, I think, because this has really forced us to talk about really awful things and communicate with each other. I mean, I tell him how he makes me feel. He may not say the right thing, but I know he tries. He's real in touch now, I think. I think he's real sensitive to a lot of my feelings. Like what makes me feel bad. So, I think it's taught us how to talk to each other more, and communicate more, and care more about each other's feelings than when we first got married.

All of this sounds too good to be true, and maybe it is. After all, many of the same couples who told us a short time ago that infertility posed problems for communication are now telling us that their marriages are stronger than ever. For example, in Chapter 1, Liz told us that she got angry at Matt because she thought his life was good and hers wasn't; now she is telling us that sharing a common problem brought the two of them closer together. Or consider another example. We heard Jeff describe a scene in which he berated Teri for exaggerating the importance of infertility, but now we hear Teri asserting that Jeff has become so much more sensitive to her feelings.

Of course, all this talk about being closer together is possibly insincere, part of an act staged by people who wanted to impress me with how great their marriages are. I don't think so, however. If people were out to impress me, their stories would have been more consistent. If they were trying to impress me with the solidity of their marriages, why would they confess their dissatisfactions so frankly? What are we to make of the apparent contradictions in the stories we are told? Should we believe the evidence that infertile wives and husbands live in different experiential worlds, or should we believe these couples when they say that infertility has brought them closer together? Are these couples together or apart? The answer, I think, is that they are both together *and* apart. There are contradictions in their accounts because there are contradictions in their experience.

American marriage is, as Lilian Rubin asserts, an alliance between intimate strangers. American husbands and wives live in different experiential worlds and apprehend virtually all aspects of their marriages from decidedly different vantage points. The infertile wives and husbands I spoke with are probably typical of most middle-class American couples. Infertility has, perhaps, brought them closer, but they are still far apart. This dramatizes just how far apart are wives' and husbands' worlds in American society and just how difficult it is for couples to realize the goal of a communicative marriage.

The couples who asserted that infertility brought them closer together by forcing them to communicate did not claim idyllic marriages. In eighteen of the couples I interviewed wives and husbands agreed that infertility increased levels of tension in their relationships. We must keep in mind that arguing, too, is a form of communication, which does not obliterate the differences in the ways husbands and wives react to infertility, but it does make husbands and wives more alive to each other's feelings. Barbara recounted:

> It brought us closer together. We communicated. I think that's been a plus, that we've been able to communicate and respect one another's opinions. There are times when I'm pretty unbearable, and I imagine he is too. That's part of a relationship. If you get along 100 percent of the time, something's the matter with the relationship.

Her husband Mike saw things in pretty much the same way:

> I think in some areas we're closer. I think our communications are in the realm of excellent. I think we talk very well together. Although I think it's put a tremendous strain on our relationship—we argue much more than we ever argued before—I still think we're much more sensitive.

Thus, it seems that while infertility introduces tension into a relationship, that which produces much of the tension—the need for people with different perspectives to work out a common course of action to deal with a common problem—may also, in the long run, make wives and husbands feel closer.

A comparison between the couples who feel that infertility has pulled them apart and those who felt it helped bring them together may be instructive here. The couples who said infertility strengthened their relationship were those who saw it as a common problem requiring communication. The couples who felt that infertility made them more distant tended to be those in which one marital partner was unwilling either to accept the problem as shared or to communicate about it. Dan, who has a low sperm count, was more affected emotionally by infertility than many other husbands. For a while, Dan was unwilling to accept Sherry's support. According to Sherry:

There has been lots of tension in the relationship, and we're just getting back together, really. Mostly what happened was that he withdrew from me, feeling his own inadequacies. It was his way of dealing with the emotional pain of it. It was like he was saying to himself, "It's my problem, and it's not her problem, and I gotta do this thing." That was real, real hard for a long time.

This example brings us back to the issue of the conflict over intimacy that is increasingly typical of American marriages. Where the husband resists his wife's demands for greater communication, infertility may stand as a barrier between them; where the husband accepts infertility as a common problem about which they need to communicate, it may unite them.

INFERTILITY AND THE EXPERIENCE OF SEX

No examination of communication and intimacy in marriage could possibly be complete without a discussion of sexuality. Studies that attempt to explore empirically the relationship between sexual satisfaction and marital satisfaction have found the two phenomena closely related. On the basis of an exhaustive survey of American couples, sociologists Philip Blumstein and Pepper Schwartz confidently assert that "a good sex life is central to a good marriage."[14]

The purported connection between good sex and good marriage is apparently related in large part to the communicative functions of sex. Psychoanalyst Aaron Stein argues that the connection between sex and marital satisfaction stems from the role sex plays in fostering marital intimacy: "It's not that sex is so vital to life, but that sex relieves tensions and provides in marriage the pleasure of closeness, the satisfaction and fulfillment of the love the couple has for one another.

The need to make love is not only a sexual one, it's a need to enjoy one another, to make contact in a concrete way."[15]

Blumstein and Schwartz note that sex serves important symbolic functions as well.[16] In American society, sex has a specific culturally assigned meaning. Sex is believed to be the consequence, the cause, and the indicator of intimacy. Good sex, in other words, for many American couples symbolizes a close relationship. In contemporary American marriages, sex serves for many as a kind of barometer of marital quality. Enjoyable sex carries with it the unspoken message that a relationship is solid and successful.

Moreover, the relationship between sex and intimacy may well differ for wives and husbands. According to Lilian Rubin, husbands often rely (sometimes exclusively) on intercourse as a means of achieving intimacy. Wives, however, often see intercourse as a natural *consequence* of intimacy achieved by other means. In other words, while husbands see sex as a source of intimacy, wives are more inclined to see it as an expression of intimacy. Needless to say, this difference of perspectives may itself be a source of tension in marriage and an obstacle to achieving intimacy.

The apparent connection between good sex and a healthy marriage would not appear to bode well for infertile couples. Many writers on infertility have argued that infertility has an especially catastrophic impact on sexual satisfaction. One review of the literature on the emotional and psychological consequences of infertility asserts that "no aspect of the couple's functioning is more affected by infertility than sexuality."[17] The wives and husbands I interviewed agreed that infertility had led to a deterioration of their sexual relationships. Only five of the twenty-two couples reported that sexual activity was as pleasurable or nearly as pleasurable as it had been before they became conscious of their problem with fertility. Because wives' and husbands' perceptions of infertility differ in so many other ways, it is interesting to note that, within couples, partners tended to agree on their evaluation of the effect of infertility on their sexual relationship.

The theme most commonly expressed by those who felt their sex lives had deteriorated involved the negative consequences of engaging in sex according to schedule. [18] Craig discussed his preoccupation with timing:

It doesn't matter whether or not you've got to get up early the next day and would really rather just sleep. Should you be having any becomes a question. Should we have intercourse tonight? Maybe it makes a difference if we have it in the morning, maybe we ought to take time off from work and go in the afternoon, or maybe it ought to be in the evening.

Paul compared the routine of scheduled sex to "boot camp." Barbara described her sexual relationship with Mike as being stressful:

The stress in the bedroom has been tremendous. We have our off nights, and we have our on nights. I've been keeping charts for three years, and it has put a damper on our sex life. Having to perform relations when you've had a wicked day at work and making a baby is the last thing on your mind or having sex for procreative purposes is sometimes frustrating.

Jim called sex a chore: "For us, it had become such a chore, it had become unpleasurable. It was not fun; it wasn't enjoyable. You did it under pressure. Whether you wanted to or not, you had to do it." For some couples, the need to plan something that "ought" to be spontaneous brought with it communication problems and emotional pain. Chip's wife Cathy recounted: "I don't remember there ever being hurt feelings before. But now all of a sudden, there were hurt feelings. I was afraid to tell him sometimes that this was a good night because I knew that he wasn't in the mood or that he was too tired. I could always tell if he was doing me a favor." Karen remembered an argument she and Brett had about scheduling sex:

This past cycle, we did have one argument where it was an "on" night and he didn't feel up to it, and I got upset because I knew that missing one month meant a whole extra month of me having to take the temperatures and take the medicines. So it was more than just not feeling up to it. If we miss this month, I have to work a whole extra month to make up for it.

Both passages I just cited can remind us of the tendency to regard infertility as the wife's problem. When Cathy says that she could tell when Chip was doing *her* a favor, she seems to be suggesting that infertility is *her* problem. She apparently appreciates the fact that Chip was willing to ignore his own desires to do her a favor. But nowhere is there a suggestion that she sees having intercourse when *she* doesn't feel like it as doing *him* a favor. In a similar manner, Karen and Brett seem to see infertility as "her work." When Brett refuses sex, Karen reacts to his refusal in terms of how she has to compensate for his unwillingness to be supportive.

The felt need to schedule sex to maximize the likelihood of conception contributed to the transforming intercourse from an end in itself into merely the means of procreation. Couples described thinking of sex as something that needs to be done rather than as something enjoyable. They often employed the term "mechanical" in their descriptions of sex.[19] Craig explained, "It's one way to turn your sex life off. Sex becomes mechanical. It becomes simply an act and something to be accomplished rather than a tender moment shared between two people who really care for each other. It doesn't become a caring thing. It's just mechanical and prescribed." Lois said that she just wanted to get it over with: "Sex was unexciting. It was too structured. I had this, 'Let's just get it over with attitude.'" Kim described sex as becoming like a job: "That was the pits. I'll say that without a shadow of hesitation. There was a point where I said, 'This is my job.'"

Most couples reported that they only engaged in sex when it was "called for." Barbara recalled: "During the fertile times it was every other day, odd days this month, even days the next month. But as far as having sex for sex's sake or sex for fun, we didn't have that much of it." For Robin, sex was just a means to have a child:

It was only a means to have a child in my book. And I really didn't care to have it any other time. Just when we had to. And when it came time to taking the temperature charts into the doctor, I put extra x's on the chart. Every time you did it, it was like, "I wonder if it's going to be this time," you know, and you're too busy trying to remember to put your legs up and the pillow under your hips or whatever your method of the month was.

Robin's comments introduce us to another theme expressed by the couples I interviewed—invasion of privacy. Robin has just described herself putting extra x's on her BBT chart so that her doctor would not know how infrequently she and her husband were engaging in intercourse during the "off season." BBT charts do more than provide the infertile couple with data on the basis of which sex is to be scheduled; they also symbolize the invasion of privacy experienced by the infertile. BBT charts are the visible reminders that sex is no longer an act that concerns two individuals alone.[20]

Debby expressed the invasion of privacy theme powerfully: "I hated it. I felt like such an idiot, not being active sexually at the right times. I felt like saying, 'It's none of your business.' It felt good getting rid of those charts." Cliff characterized the BBT routine as embarrassing: "It was a pain in the butt. You know, you sit down and take the temperature and mark it down on the chart. Sometimes you'd do it, and sometimes you'd forget. And I think telling the doctor what was going on, you were embarrassed."

A final factor contributing to the negative evaluation of sex among infertile couples is the fact that the sexual act itself may only remind one of one's infertility. Peg said: "You would get very romantically inclined and everything, and then you'd start making love. And, all of a sudden, in the back of my mind, I'm saying, 'Well is this going to make me pregnant?'" For Rachel also intercourse was a reminder of failure: "It always reminded me of something we couldn't do. Every time we had sex it was a reminder that, 'Well, we probably won't get pregnant this time.'"

Given the purported relationship between sexual satisfaction and marital satisfaction, it would seem reasonable to assume that a spoiled sexual life would lead to more general marital problems for infertile couples. Surprisingly, the couples in my sample who reported that infertility had a severe negative impact on their sexual lives were *not* more likely to report that infertility had a negative impact upon their relationship. Approximately half the couples in both groups felt that infertility had brought them closer together. How is it that sexual satisfaction seems unrelated to marital satisfaction or felt intimacy among the infertile? I think the answer to this question lies in the fact that the experience of infertility transforms the symbolic meaning of sex.

As we have seen, American couples often regard satisfying sex as the symbol of a healthy relationship. The context in which infertile couples engage in intercourse strips sex of its implications of intimacy, making it instead a chore, a means to an end, a mechanical act. But, at the same time, infertility may let sex "off the hook." Because sexual problems—even those that may have existed prior to a couple defining themselves as infertile—can be attributed to infertility, sex may lose some of its status as the symbol of a satisfying relationship.

Unsatisfying sex may also prompt the infertile to develop means of promoting and expressing intimacy outside sexual relations. Debra Kaufman's study of Jewish women who have recently converted to Orthodox Judaism may be instructive here, although it would seem at first glance to have no connection to infertility.[21] Kaufman discusses the newly Orthodox women's responses to laws of *niddah* that declare a woman ritually impure during and immediately after her menstrual cycle and forbid intercourse during that period. Niddah appears archaic and demeaning to women, but Kaufman gives it a feminist reading. Far from complaining about the unfairness or the restrictiveness of niddah, many women spoke of it favorably, saying that the two-week period of enforced sexual abstinence has actually strengthened their marriages by preventing their husbands from relying so exclusively on sex as a means of communication. According to these women, niddah has improved their marital relationships by forcing their husbands to learn new forms of communication.

Infertility may, for some couples, have a similar paradoxical effect. Infertility, too, inhibits the ability of sex to serve as *the* foundation of marital intimacy. We may, perhaps, speculate that, in some cases, the ruinous effect of infertility on sexual satisfaction actually strengthens relationships by forcing infertile couples to develop new ways to communicate. Blumstein and Schwartz have found that husbands' ability to be tender and expressive is an important factor contributing to the stability of marriage.[22] If infertility leads husbands to improve their skills at building intimacy, then it could indirectly improve marital stability.

At the same time that the experience of infertility removes from many couples the possibility of using sex as a resource for constructing intimacy, it may ironically supply them with another: the shared experience of infertility itself. The sense of being "in this thing together" characterizes many infertile couples; this can enhance communication and thus strengthen their sense of intimacy.

To conclude, the effects of infertility on communication and intimacy within marriage are not clearcut. Infertility may threaten intimacy by dramatizing for husbands and wives just how different their experiential worlds are and just how difficult it is for them to construct a shared reality. Infertility can also threaten intimacy by disabling sexuality as a viable resource for constructing intimacy. But infertility, to the extent that couples perceive it as a shared crisis to be overcome together, can also supply a source of intimacy.

Infertility has an impact on communication and intimacy, not only because of the inherent characteristics of infertility as a health problem, but also because tensions regarding intimacy and communication already exist in American marriages. Infertility becomes an issue of communication and intimacy because conflict over communication and intimacy are built into the current structure of American marriage. Given this fact, any crisis that confronts American couples presents itself—at least, in part—as a crisis of intimacy.

SIX

A SECRET STIGMA
Interaction with the Fertile World

A major theme in the sociological literature on chronic illness and disability concerns the strain that often characterizes relationships between sufferers and "normals."[1] Chronic illness and disability might interfere with everyday social interaction for several reasons: they render the sufferer unable to behave in an acceptable manner; they prevent the sufferer from meeting the expectations of others; or their very visibility casts a pall over the interaction. Sufferers from chronic illness and disability often feel either that they have been stigmatized or, if their condition is unknown to others, that they would be stigmatized if others found them out.[2]

INFERTILITY AS A SOCIAL STIGMA

Sociologist Charlene Miall has noted that the infertile, like the chronically ill and disabled, see their condition as stigmatized by society at large. The infertile women Miall interviewed complained about three widely held attitudes they saw as stigmatizing: the belief that the causes of infertility are psychological rather than physical, the association of infertility with sexual incompetence, and the assumption that infertility is basically a women's problem.[3]

126

The medical history of infertility is replete with examples of infertile people, especially women, being held responsible for their own condition. In 1883, physician Matthew J. Duncan questioned whether sterility should be treated at all because infertile women were clearly genetically inferior and should therefore not be encouraged to propagate. In 1924 Donald Macomber wrote in the *Journal of the American Medical Association* that a major cause of sterility was "poor hygiene" among adolescent girls; one aspect of poor hygiene Macomber particularly noted was the failure of girls to stay in bed during their menstrual cycles. In 1956, Sommers H. Sturgis, in his presidential address to the American Society for the Study of Sterility, was quite explicit in connecting sterility and women's pursuit of higher education.[4]

In a review of the contemporary scholarly and professional literature on infertility, Margarete Sandelowski, a nurse and writer on medical themes, suggests that authors are still holding women responsible for their own infertility.[5] Sandelowski argues that—by emphasizing the effects of delayed childbearing on the ability to conceive, the hazards of the work place in causing infertility, and the role of sexually transmitted diseases in giving rise to infertility—contemporary writers are leaving the impression that women have brought infertility upon themselves through deserting traditional role expectations for women.

Although the incomplete state of the crosscultural literature on infertility does not permit me to state unequivocally that the tendency to blame the infertile for their own misfortune is found in all cultures, it is certainly found in many. In 1945, anthropologist Clellan Stearns Ford was able to enumerate twenty-eight societies in which infertility was "despised, ridiculed, or pitied." Studies have shown that people throughout the world—blacks, Mormons, and others in the United States; Polish, Serbian, and Jewish peasants in Europe; numerous societies in Africa—look down upon the infertile. Among the Ashanti of Africa, an infertile man is called "wax penis." The South American Cagaba refer to an infertile woman as a "mule."[6]

In this chapter, I examine infertile couples' views of the fertile world's perceptions of infertility. I also explore the ways in which the fertile world's perceptions of infertility—and the perception of those perceptions by the infertile—influence the way in which infertile and fertile people interact.

During the course of my conversation with Debby, I asked her if she felt that people discriminate against her because she is infertile. She answered with a catalogue of the ways in which the fertile discriminate against the infertile:

> By insensitivity, by maybe taking their fertility for granted, and by being incredibly nosey. "So when are you going to have kids?" How can you ask that of somebody? I think they discriminate by making light of the problem. I don't have terminal cancer, but this ain't fun. "Adopt and you'll get pregnant," that little piece of bullshit. As if this is just an emotional situation. Endometriosis is not emotional; endometriosis is real. And just sort of making light of something that affects people. Discrimination is there when you go to family picnics, or those kinds of things, where it's just assumed that you're a family.

Debby has made three charges against the fertile world, charges repeated by many other people I spoke to. First, she accused the fertile world of intruding into the private lives of the infertile by asking questions about topics that were none of their business. Second, she criticized the fertile for treating the plight of the infertile as if trivial and inconsequential. Finally, she charged them with assuming that having children is the normal state of affairs, easily attainable by everyone who aspires to it.

A number of the people I interviewed, mostly wives, raised the issue of "invasion of privacy." People talked about their resentment over the constant pressure they felt to make public their private suffering. They complained, for example, about being constantly asked by people who did not know they were infertile whether they had any children. This question, although asked innocently, was just one

more reminder of infertility in a round of life already too full of
reminders.

Not only those who were unaware of a couple's infertility asked
painful questions. Friends and relatives who knew a couple was pursuing treatment would often ask—sometimes out of concern, sometimes out of curiosity—questions that would make an individual feel
like an outsider and a failure. Lois was particularly sensitive to the
invasion of her privacy by people who asked her if she was pregnant
yet:

> Finally, I got to the point where I just said, "Well, when I am,
> I'll let you know." Because it was like, after surgery, that was all
> I ever heard, "Well, are you pregnant yet?" I felt like saying,
> "Don't you think if I was, I'd have told you?" Such crudeness to
> me is very rude, to even ask anybody. I mean, I know they were
> saying it kind of fun like, but to me it wasn't fun. You know, it
> wasn't anything that I could joke about.

Many people I spoke to also complained that fertile people acted as
if their infertility were a small and relatively easy problem to solve.
To be told that something that preoccupied them day and night was
not really very important was especially painful to the infertile
wives. Again, Lois was particularly attuned to insensitive remarks of
this nature: "We know another couple, and she was somewhat supportive, but I always felt as if she was kind of blasé about it a little bit.
You know, 'It'll happen, you're so young,' is always what I heard.
'You're so young.' Well, what does it matter what age you are? The
point is I want it now. It doesn't matter if I'm 60 or if I'm too old—I
want it to be now."

It was equally painful to hear people suggest that the problem
commanding so much time and emotional energy actually had a very
simple solution. Dee complained about some advice she received
from friends: "They would just kind of like say, 'Well, why don't you
do IVF?' They would just simplify it when it wasn't that simple, and

I would get angry. Or 'Why don't you go on a cruise?' Or 'Why don't you just relax? And then you'll get pregnant.'"

But perhaps the most painful comments of all were those that implied one was actually lucky to be infertile. Jean, who had adopted a baby, described an upsetting incident that occurred at a baby shower: "I was at one baby shower recently where a friend of mine, as they were going around everybody telling their labor and delivery stories, spoke up and said, 'Jean had it easy. She just had to drive downtown.' Like that was all I had to do." Carol described how she felt upon being told that she was better off without kids:

> This girl that I know hurt my feelings one time because she was pregnant and she probably wasn't too happy about it. It was her third in three years or something like that. And I was saying it was really nice, and she said, "Why is it always the women with no children that think it's so wonderful when you get pregnant?" And I felt like she hit me in the stomach.

Far and away the most common complaint about the fertile was that their actions and comments seemed to reflect a total unawareness of the existence of infertility or the pain it causes. According to the couples I spoke with, most people seemed totally oblivious to the possibility that constant references to pregnancy, childbirth, and babies could cause others to suffer deeply. As a place where one frequently encountered casual acquaintances, work was particularly likely to be the scene of such innocent attacks. Tom told of the strains of social interaction at work: "There've been a couple times when people at work have been extremely insensitive, not through any fault of their own, just not knowing my condition. They would come up and say, 'Well, guess what we just found out—we're pregnant again. It's our third kid, you know, and we didn't even want the second one,' and things like that." Robin recounted an incident at work that really "got to her": "One of the foremen where I was working came out, and his wife had been ill. I said to him, 'Is she feeling better? How's she doing?' And he said, 'Oh, yeah, she's fine. Nothing that nine months won't cure,' as he merrily walked out of the place. I went outside, and I think I cried for an hour that day."

Many wives and a few husbands reported that informal social gatherings could be quite unpleasant. Jean commented that, even after adopting a child, she still found it difficult to deal with baby showers: "Baby showers can still bother me because it's a kind of ritual at baby showers where at a certain time during the gathering all the women have to tell their labor and delivery stories." Teri reported problems handling apparently innocent get-togethers:

> There's been a couple of little parties given for the women, like cosmetic parties where somebody comes in and sells makeup. One was to decorate your home, and they sold all kinds of things to decorate your house and stuff. The last one I went to was the last one I'm going to ever, and it was awful. It was just like this room full of women, and every single one of them is a mother, and all they did was talk about it. Everything from getting your figure back in shape after delivery, to breast feeding, to babysitters. It was horrible for me. I hated it. And I just said, "I'm not going to subject myself to those situations anymore."

In the episodes I have just recounted, no one has actually told someone who is infertile that he or she is deviant or abnormal. But my respondents did recount a few instances where they were actually told face to face that people regarded their childless state as abnormal. Mary described a scene in which old acquaintances actually berated her for not having children:

> We had been married about four years. We walked into a bar one night, and acquaintances of ours sat down and suddenly decided to have this long talk with us. Where were we getting off being married four years and not having any children? Didn't we know that money wasn't everything? Why were we so money hungry, and why was I being such a bitch to my husband, not giving him the children that he rightly deserved?

131

Earlier, we heard Debby speak about discrimination against the infertile, but if we take discrimination to mean *deliberate* action taken against persons or groups because of certain characteristics they possess, then the term "discrimination" is a little misleading. The main source of unsatisfactory interaction in these stories does not seem to be attitudes on the part of others that the infertile are inferior because of their condition. Rather, the chief source of dissatisfaction is the failure of others to acknowledge the seriousness of infertility. The infertile wives and husbands I interviewed used the term "insensitive" to describe people who were ignorant of infertility's devastating effects on identity.

Most people I spoke to are quite aware that many comments they have found painful or offensive were offered innocently. And they are aware that their infertility leads them to take offense at comments they might otherwise let pass. Jim is one husband who spoke to this point: "A passing comment would be meaningless ordinarily, but it would just hit the wrong way. And I would be upset with whoever said it because it would upset Mary. I'd say, 'What's the matter with you? Isn't it obvious that was the wrong thing to say?'"

In many cases, the insensitive people described in the infertile's stories are not even aware that the person they have offended is infertile. In fact, the most hurtful comments reported above were made by those who assumed that the person they spoke to was not infertile but *voluntarily* childless.

FELT STIGMA AND ENACTED STIGMA

It is important to point out in this context how infertility is distinguished from the most obvious examples of disability and chronic illness that spring to mind—it is *invisible*. Unlike paraplegics or the blind, the infertile possess a *secret stigma*; they display no obvious stigmatizing features, and it is relatively easy for them to pass as normal. The infertile have a condition neither visibly discrediting nor obviously discreditable. Unlike those with epilepsy, for example, who must be concerned that an inopportune seizure might reveal their stigmatizing condition to others, the infertile are relatively free to keep their stigma secret.[7] Debby contrasted the experience of the infertile with that of the deaf: "When I walk into a store and look at baby clothes, nobody knows that they're not for me. Nobody knows that I'm dying to buy that for my own kid. Nobody knows that I'm lusting after maternity clothes. But if I would go into a store and talk in sign language, it would be clear that I couldn't pass."

Considering how easy it is to pass as normal, it is striking that the people I spoke to felt the stigma of infertility so strongly. Sociologist Graham Scambler has made a distinction between *enacted stigma* that stems from intentional discrimination against the stigmatized and *felt stigma*; there the stigmatized feel shame because they internalized societal evaluations of their condition, and, as a result, they sense their failure to live up to the standards of normality. In their study of epileptics, Scambler and Hopkins found that family members played an important role in fostering felt stigma by sending clear messages to the sufferer concerning how people would react if they found out about his or her condition. It would seem that for these infertile couples, as for the epileptics studied by Scambler, felt stigma was the source of more anguish than enacted stigma.[8]

As we have seen in Chapter 3 the heart of the experience of infertility appears to lie in the inability to proceed with one's life according to life course norms that are both reinforced by others and accepted as valid by the affected individual. Given this pervasive sense of failure, especially among infertile wives, it is easy to understand how the world can appear as a place full of discrediting messages about self, even absent deliberate attempts on the part of fertile people to stigmatize the infertile. Fertile people promote the stigmatization of the infertile not so much by deliberately discriminating as by promoting a definition of normality that excludes the infertile.

These observations draw our attention to the crucial importance of self-labeling in shaping the experience of infertility.[9] Many discussions of stigmatized health conditions—in fact, many general discussions of stigma and labeling—have implicitly assumed that the labeled individual merely responds passively to a negative label imposed by others. A number of scholars have rejected this assumption, arguing that those who are targets of a label take an active role, either by resisting or accepting the label.[10] Even these writers, however, generally assume that self-labeling must necessarily occur in the context of labeling attempts by others or in the context of fear that such attempts may be forthcoming.

In her discussion of self-labeling processes in mental illness, sociologist Peggy Thoits has taken a different tack; she argues that self-labeling may take place when individuals recognize in themselves deviations from "expression norms" to which they themselves subscribe.[11] In a similar manner, my analysis suggests that the major source of stigma among the infertile is the feeling that they have failed to live up to norms in which they strongly believe.

THE STIGMA OF INFERTILITY IN CROSSCULTURAL PERSPECTIVE

While it appears that infertility has been associated with social stigma in most—if not all—societies, it is probably not the case that infertility has been a secret stigma in most societies. The stigma of infertility can only be secret in contemporary American society because motives exist for not wanting children. The infertile people I spoke to were often assumed to be voluntarily childless. Mary's acquaintances berated her, not because they knew she couldn't have children, but because they mistakenly thought she didn't want children; she was criticized, not for being physically imperfect, but for being selfish.

In most traditional societies, voluntary childlessness is virtually unknown. Among such peoples as the Tiv or the Ganda, where a woman's social status depends almost exclusively on her achievement of the status of motherhood, the idea that someone might not want children seems virtually unthinkable. In traditional societies throughout the world—the Taiwanese and the Thai in Asia, the

Dogon and the Ganda in Africa, the Tlingit, the Iroquois, and the Tzeltal of the Americas—the desire for children is assumed by most people to be universal. In such societies, there is no secret to the stigma of infertility. If a woman does not have children, people assume she is infertile. If a woman in a Greek village is not pregnant within a year of her marriage, people begin to gossip about her inability to have children. If a Taiwanese woman has not become pregnant within several months of her marriage, her mother-in-law will begin to ask blunt questions about her menstrual cycle.[12]

Infertility can only be a secret stigma in societies where women are believed to have reasonable motives for not wanting to become mothers. The development of such motives is apparently related to industrialization.[13] Because it alters the cost/benefits ratio of having children and because it at least offers women a glimpse of the possibility of rewards found in roles that do not involve childbearing, industrialization makes the idea of not wanting children plausible.

Although conclusive data on this point are not available, my best guess is that, in American society, infertility evolved from a public stigma into a secret stigma during the second half of the nineteenth century. I base this guess primarily on demographic data concerning the incidence of childlessness. The percentage of married American women who reached their forty-fifth birthday without bearing a child increased slowly but perceptibly from 1885 to 1910.[14] Childlessness rates for women forty-five and older who have ever been married, continued to rise until 1950, when they began to drop.[15] In recent years childlessness rates have begun to rise again. The most plausible interpretation of these data seems to be that most childlessness before the 1880s was due to infertility and that the increase in childlessness after that time was due to a rise in voluntary childlessness. Fluctuations in childlessness rates during the twentieth century appear primarily the result of changes in the incidence of voluntary childlessness as people responded to variations in economic opportunities and social values.

If this interpretation is correct, then, by the early twentieth century, most childlessness was voluntary. When sociologists Robert and Helen Lynd conducted their famous Middletown studies of Muncie, Indiana, in the 1920s and 1930s, clearly the majority of Middletown residents assumed that most childless couples had chosen their childless state and turned their backs on moral obligation.[16] Thus, infertility, once very public, had become invisible.

As infertility became invisible, it was transformed from a public experience into a private one. As a result of this transformation, a sense of loneliness became a core component of the experience of infertility. The infertile, and especially infertile wives, bear the burden of a suffering that they often believe no one else shares or understands. I do not intend to argue that the invisibility of infertility has made it any harder to bear than it may have been at other times and in other places. It is not easy to say whether private suffering is better or worse than public humiliation. It is clear, however, that the experience of a visible stigma differs significantly from the experience of a secret stigma. I wish to emphasize that the rise of voluntary childlessness has fundamentally altered the experience of infertility by making that experience more private than it once was.

TELLING AND NOT TELLING

People afflicted with a discrediting stigma must constantly confront the task of coping with the spoiled interaction that results from other people's awareness of their condition. Those with a discreditable stigma are often preoccupied with strategies for preventing others from becoming aware of their condition. For those with a secret stigma, deciding whom and how much to tell about their condition becomes a central concern.

Of the couples I spoke to, all but one had told their parents about their infertility. All but one wife and four husbands had told at least a few close friends about their situation. But almost no one made it a practice to reveal their infertility routinely to casual acquaintances. Some people confessed to being ashamed to disclose their secret to others. Debby referred to confessing one's infertility as "an incredible admission":

> I feel it's admitting some massive fault. Like telling you that there is a door, and you can just see inside that it's all screwed up. Like I'm not a regular person. It's an incredible admission to say that my sperm count is low or that my tubes are blocked. It's something we assume all our lives. It's like saying something is real wrong with you.

Others kept quiet because they were leery of the responses they might receive if they "went public." Craig said:

> We don't share the information with other people, simply because we're ill at ease with it. It's not something that's easily handled. It's not like saying, "Oh, gee, I have an infected tooth; I'd better go to the dentist." It's something that still has somewhat of a taboo in my mind to talk about in general with people. Mostly because I'm still leery of crude comments, of having my feelings hurt. I'm reluctant to talk about it with just about anyone in the general population. Unless it's to achieve a specific goal, a purpose.

Thus, people withheld information from others because they both felt the stigma of infertility deeply and feared the social consequences of revealing their stigma to others. There is nothing very surprising in the fact that the people I interviewed were reluctant to talk about their situation with others. Their reasons for keeping infertility in the closet seem sensible. The literature on social stigma would lead one to believe that anyone able to keep a stigma secret would have strong motivations to take advantage of that ability.

Given that infertile couples have some powerful reasons for hiding their infertility, we need to ask why anyone would ever choose to tell people. Sociologists Robert Gramling and Craig J. Forsythe have pointed out that people sometimes do have sound reasons for drawing attention to a stigmatized condition. Someone might choose to "advertise" stigma, according to Gramling and Forsythe, to elicit special consideration. I have already drawn attention to the loneliness of infertility. People may confess their infertility out of a need for support and social validation. In addition, they may find that keeping infertility a secret is simply too much of a psychic burden to bear. In any case, the decision to tell involves a risk, because—as we have already seen—fertile friends may not prove supportive and understanding.[17]

Some couples told others to keep people from making insensitive remarks on the assumption that they were childless by choice. Teri decided to tell at least a few close friends and relatives so that she would not be burdened with having to fend off a lot of "stupid questions." Teri's husband Jeff agrees that telling people was a good idea:

> She's told our friends, which is ok, because a lot of our friends have given us a lot of grief about waiting as long as we did to have children. Because they had children, they said, "Don't wait so long." And then, after we started trying and weren't successful, of course, that kind of kidding really went to the heart quite a bit, especially with my wife. She would get all agitated with people, and sometimes she would say some inappropriate thing. So it's good that all of our friends have been told.

Others told to keep people from getting "the wrong idea" about them. Karen told friends so that they would make allowances for her bad moods: "It's just something that I talk about because I need to talk about it. I need for other people to understand when I get really moody, which I do." Rachel felt it necessary to tell people at work so that they would not misconstrue her frequent absences: "I ended up having to tell most of the people that I work with that we're having fertility problems because, when you go to the doctor every month, people think either you're having an affair with your doctor or that there's something deathly wrong with you."

Gramling and Forsythe mention another reason for admitting to stigma: to avoid a more serious stigma. Teri and Jeff told people about their infertility problems to avoid being chastised for *choosing* to be childless. Karen told people about her trouble conceiving as a means of accounting for her moodiness. Rachel went public about infertility to prevent her work mates from drawing the conclusion that she was either seriously ill or feigning illness out of some ulterior motive. In many of these cases, telling about infertility was perceived as a decision to admit the lesser of two stigmas. Some writers on the subject of deviance have distinguished between "accidental deviance," over which an individual is presumed to have no control, and "deliberate deviance," which is presumed intentional.[18] Forced to confess to either accidental or deliberate deviance, people generally chose the former.

RELATIONSHIPS WITH FRIENDS

As we have seen, invisibility did not lessen the salience of infertility in everyday life. Although their infertility was often a secret to others, the infertile couples I spoke to, especially the wives, nonetheless felt that stigma acutely. And their consciousness of the need to account for their behavior to others heightened their sense that a chasm of experience lay between themselves and the fertile world. This chasm of experience made them feel radically different from all fertile people. Mary eloquently expressed this feeling of being different: "The feeling of being different from all of my friends who had children and got pregnant with them. And knowing that they would never understand where I was coming from. There's always going to be a difference between us." Debby described infertility as a lonely state: "It's real lonely. If you don't find other people, it's real lonely. You feel like you are the only one on earth who could feel this way."

Infertile couples' relationships with friends and relatives were inevitably colored by their conviction that people who had not experienced infertility could not really understand the way they felt. Martha didn't see the point of talking to others too much about her infertility:

> The only other people I've found that I've been able to talk to about it are other people who have gone through it. People who have had children seem to think that. . . . I don't know, I just don't feel they understand until it happens to them. I'll explain the situation to other people, but I won't get into real emotional things or anything—only with other people who have gone through the same thing.

Many people I spoke to said that maintaining relationships with people who had children had become trying for them.[19] Mike remarked that it had become difficult for him and Barbara to sustain relationships with friends who had children: "We haven't lost any friends, but I think somehow relationships change. A lot of our friends have kids, and some of them camp together, and I think we would be doing things more with them if we had our kids." Being around friends with children was difficult, because—even more than strangers—these friends constantly but unintentionally remind the infertile of their exclusion from the fertile world. Cliff was also bothered by being around friends who couldn't talk about anything but their kids: "Some of our friends, not intentionally, would talk about their kids an awful lot, and they knew that we couldn't have any children. And I think that was bothering us psychologically. I don't think they did it intentionally, but it did bother us."

As we have seen, infertile couples, especially infertile wives, often strongly sense that they are outsiders in a fertile world. One of the most poignant reminders of one's exclusion from normalcy came when childless friends announced that they were pregnant. When this happened, couples often expressed the feeling that they had been betrayed. Such events dramatized even more than most others the sense of being an outsider. According to Liz, "The hardest ones were the people who didn't have kids and who I didn't think were going to have kids. You would think, 'Well, this couple isn't going to have kids, and we can keep going out with them.' These could be life-long friends. And, all of a sudden, she'd get pregnant. Those were the ones."

While the people I have been quoting were critical of their friends for always talking about children and babies or for not minding their own business, some wives also criticized friends who took pains to avoid confronting them with reminders of infertility. Cathy said that many of her friends were afraid to bring up the subject of her infer-tility: "Everyone felt that the less they brought it up, the better for me. They didn't want to bring up a sore subject." Sally got angry at a pregnant friend who didn't think she was strong enough to take the news: "The only time I can remember being angry at someone who told me she was pregnant, she told me when she was about four months. And the way she told me was, 'I didn't really want to tell you because I was afraid you would feel bad.'"

Couples used different strategies for dealing with fertile friends. Perhaps the most popular strategy was simply to avoid being around friends with children. Barbara said that she and Mike often em-ployed this tactic: "We developed friendships with people who didn't have children. It seemed easier that way than to deal with people who had kids. We maintained some relationships with people with kids, but they weren't in depth. They seemed to be more superficial. You know, How are the kids doing? How's the job? How's the weather? How's the house coming?—and not much about kids." Ac-cording to Cliff, he and Peg went so far as to contemplate moving to a new area just to get away from fertile friends: "I think we just burned ourselves out to a point where we decided that we better move to someplace where we would meet couples that didn't have any kids. It was easier to be with them than it was to go with somebody that had young kids."

Other couples tried to preserve friendships by hiding their feel-ings.[20] Because they did not feel it appropriate to burden their friends with their personal problems, these couples took a "grin-and-bear-it" approach to dealing with fertile friends. Carol would not let on to her fertile friends how painful it was to be around them: "I had several friends who waited a long time before having children. And as, one by one, they started to have their children, it would just be hard. But I never dropped friends because of it, and I never avoided them because of it. I felt bad because that's one more who's doing what I'd like to do."

Mary felt that the best way for her and Jim to deal with fertile friends was to be as "up front" about their feelings as they could be:

> We talked to anybody and everybody who would listen to us about infertility. We were very, very vocal. So it was kind of an obsession with us. All we talked about for two years was our infertility problem. With all of my friends, eventually we worked through any difficulties that we had because of infertility. Sometimes, it meant being apart from each other for a couple of months, maybe, while they were getting toward the end of their pregnancies. I couldn't deal with that particular part of it. But, it was a sit-down thing: "OK, you're getting to the point in your pregnancy where I just can't look at you without great pain. I need to be away from you until after the baby is born." So everything was up front.

But whatever approach a couple took to the question of how to deal with fertile friends, the chasm of experience remained. And, while many friendships survived, few were unaffected by the perception on the part of the infertile that that chasm was impossible to bridge.

DEALING WITH RELATIVES

When they interacted with relatives, the couples I interviewed faced many of the same problems they confronted when dealing with friends. Family members, just as friends, can come to seem like representatives of the fertile world whose very presence drives home the intolerability of infertility. Janet found it hard to be around her sister: "I have a tendency to be jealous. My sister just got married two years ago. Their anniversary is this month, and she just had a little boy. He's maybe seven months old now. I was jealous of her. I made excuses not to go to see her at the hospital because I felt bad."

The people I spoke with often accused their families of the same kinds of insensitivities they complained of when they spoke of the fertile world in general. They charged family members with underestimating the seriousness of the problem and offering simple solutions in a complex situation. Liz's mother thought that if Liz would just relax, things would take care of themselves: "Well, she always felt that if I would just relax and forget the whole thing, then I would get pregnant. That was Mom's philosophy. You know, she didn't really understand that there were any medical problems that weren't caused by nerves." Like fertile people in general, family members tended to assume that pregnancy is normal and easy to achieve and that the only reason for not having children is lack of desire. Jean recalled some comments made by members of Rick's family:

Rick's family was really hot and heavy into when were we going to have a family. My family wasn't quite as bad along that line. Rick's sister, in particular. Every time we'd see her, she would say, "Well, if you don't get pregnant soon, I'm going to have a garage sale and sell all my baby stuff that I've been saving for you. It's taking up too much space." So it got to the point where we'd just avoid his side of the family.

This is not to say that no people I spoke with saw their families as supportive. Mary saw her mother as being someone who "really understood" and was grateful for her support: "My mother had an infertility problem. My mother's sister had an infertility problem. My mother lost several pregnancies, so there was a real awareness of the kind of grief that we were going through. They were nothing but supportive." Robin found some family members more supportive than others:

> I have a younger sister who hadn't experienced infertility or anything like that, but she was always good. It was like she read a book on the proper things to say to your infertile, married sister. I always said she should write the book. But she always knew the right things to say. And after my mother would totally blow something, my sister would kind of be able to calm things over for me so I wouldn't go back and blow up at my mother for being so narrow-minded.

Many people I talked with reported a great deal of continuity between their relationships with family members before and after infertility. Those who had good relationships with their families before infertility seemed much more likely to see family members as supportive. Those who did not have such good relationships with their families before infertility tended to see them as less supportive. Although Liz's mother did not always understand where Liz was coming from, Liz was glad to have her around to talk to: "I was angry at just about everyone. But my mother, I could tell her that I was angry." Stuart's relationship with his parents had soured long before infertility became an issue: "My family's a joke. Her family always kept their opinion to themselves. My family was always out with an opinion that was never worth listening to." Richard too saw continuity between the before and after periods: "I don't believe there's been any change as far as our parents are concerned. There have been a couple of ignorant remarks here and there that hurt, but, before the infertility, those remarks were there from certain family members so that hasn't changed."

Couples were often unsure about whether they would prefer family members to give them "space" to work out their problems on their own or whether they would prefer family members to show support by being more actively involved. They seemed aware that it was not easy for parents and others to decide how much involvement was enough and how much was too much. Peg appreciated her parents' and in-laws' apparent decisions not to become too involved:

> They never really said a lot to us. My mom was very supportive. . . . When I had the surgery, they came out and my mom stayed with me for a week until I got back on my feet. She knew that we wanted more children, but she didn't push it by saying, "Don't you think you ought to go for more tests." I guess she just figured it was our lives and that we would do what we thought best.

Stuart sometimes wishes Lois's parents would take a more active role than they did:

> My in-laws are almost to the point where I wish they would ask some questions, but they just don't butt in, period. They don't. If you don't offer, they don't ask. So if you want them to know something, you have to offer the information. And sometimes it's annoying. Sometimes you wonder if they care. They do care, but they go to the extreme in making sure they don't get involved in your marriage.

People seemed more willing to make allowances for family members than they would be for friends or acquaintances. Many laughed off remarks made by parents or siblings that might have been seen as "insensitive" had they been made by nonfamily members. Jim did not take his parents' inability to really comprehend what he and Mary were going through as evidence of their insensitivity: "My parents were not unfeeling: they were just unaware of how deep our feelings were, Mary's especially." Mary also recognized how difficult it was for family members to know what to do and say, and she expressed a willingness to "give them some slack": "Our families had a hard time not knowing what to say, and we had to allow for them to make mistakes, too." Mary appreciated the fact that Jim's mother tried to be supportive:

Jim's parents are in their seventies. They're just from a generation that doesn't talk about that kind of stuff openly, and they would try very hard to be supportive, but in a very quiet, quiet way. They always let us know that they were there for us if there was anything that they could do. Jim's mother was always there with her cheery little stories. They were aggravating, and I didn't like them, but I knew what she was trying to do.

Although the couples I spoke to did seem more willing to make allowances for family members than they were for friends, they still conveyed a feeling that a rift existed between themselves and representatives of the fertile world, regardless of whether these representatives were related. People appreciated attempts on the part of parents, siblings, and others to be supportive, but they still harbored the conviction that people who had not experienced infertility could not really understand what they were going through.

THE NEED FOR SUPPORT

Thus, the invisibility of infertility reinforced the sense of otherness felt by the infertile, especially infertile wives. In spite of its invisibility, infertility remained salient. Questions of whom to tell and when, questions of how much to disclose, were often on people's minds. Their feeling of failure led infertile wives to see themselves as fundamentally different from fertile friends, relatives, and others.

This feeling of separateness, of being radically different from everyone else, made some wives feel as if they were going crazy. No one, sometimes not even their husbands, seemed able to understand how infertility was affecting them. No one seemed able to comprehend why they were making such a big deal about something they ought to be taking in their stride. This perceived lack of comprehension of their reactions to infertility made some infertile wives wonder if there really was something wrong with them. Liz said that she often felt this way: "At times I felt that I really must be irrational because everybody else always thought it. I mean, I felt Matt was in the same situation, and yet he didn't react the same way at all."

Sociologist Peggy Thoits has suggested that a major function of support groups is that the presence of others with similar feelings validates one's own feelings and allows one to feel like less of an "emotional deviant." Another sociologist, Thomasina Borkman, has pointed out that it is incorrect to assume—just because a sufferer has social networks of family and friends—that these network members are perceived by this sufferer as supportive. Even people surrounded by family and friends can still feel lonely. Family and friends, Borkman says, are often guided by "folk knowledge" that leads them to stigmatize the person they are trying to help. Self-help groups allow sufferers to augment their social networks with members who, because they share the sufferer's problem, are capable of offering real support.[21]

Wives who discovered Resolve experienced tremendous gratification from knowing that other people out there had similar feelings. Cathy found the Resolve newsletters especially helpful:

> Their newsletters were an unbelievable help to me. And I'm sure that part of that stemmed from the fact that Chip wasn't able to communicate with me on the level that I needed. I needed feelings, and that's what he can't express. And so reading the articles, somebody else could put into words what I couldn't put into words. Or I could see myself in that article and say, "So I'm not going crazy." So the newsletter was the biggest help to me.

For many wives, Resolve became a locus for the formation of new primary groups—made up of people who could "really understand"—to replace the fertile friends around whom they no longer felt comfortable. According to Rachel, she and Tom replaced their network of fertile friends with friends from Resolve:

> It was really hard because, when we started trying to have kids, it was about the same time that all of our friends started

trying to have kids. And I just felt really, really awful around all of our fertile friends, who were either pregnant or were having kids. It really pulled us apart from all of our fertile friends. At the same point, I ended up getting very involved in Resolve. And it's amazing, but you talk to other people that are infertile, and you feel sort of instantly close to them. So, very gradually, our network of friends shifted from fertile to infertile people. We still have some fertile friends but not as many and not as close as before we found we were infertile.

While these wives saw Resolve as an antidote to feelings of being apart from the fertile world, it may also be the case that participation in Resolve can heighten the sense that they have a secret stigma. Participation in an in-group often leads to a magnified feeling of being different from the out-group. Participants in a support group may be encouraged to see themselves as the type of people who need the group's support. Thus, we should be wary of simply asserting that people came to Resolve because they needed support. We must be open also to the possibility that involvement with Resolve led people to reinterpret their experience so that they regarded the fertile world as being less supportive than they might have felt it to be before they became involved. And, if membership in Resolve does affect the way people interpret their experiences of infertility, we must be careful not to overgeneralize from my sample, in which Resolve members are well represented, to the infertile population as a whole.

The infertile, of course, are not the only sufferers in American society who turn to support groups for help. The United States is now witnessing a "self-help revolution."[22] One journalist estimates that approximately fifteen million people attend support group meetings in the United States during any given week.[23] This is not the place to offer a detailed analysis of the phenomenal growth of the self-help movement. It is worth pointing out, however, that this phenomenon seems to indicate that loneliness on the part of sufferers is quite common in contemporary America.

Some husbands, predominantly but not exclusively those who

themselves had reproductive impairments, also found great satisfaction in discovering people who they saw as similar to themselves. Rick described the way he reacted when he encountered someone like himself at a Resolve meeting:

> I finally found this guy who had the same scars as me, and I just latched on to that guy like you wouldn't believe. And then he said, "That guy over there's got scars, and he's got scars, and he's got scars." And we all got together there at the meeting. I went out of there, and I said, "Alright, somebody knows the shit I've been going through." And that's when it started with Resolve.

But, although Rick and Dan found Resolve immensely helpful, many husbands did not feel the need to get involved. Nineteen wives said that they felt a strong need for support, but only eight husbands said they felt this way. Jeff was typical of the husbands who had no desire to join a self-help group: "I don't think I'll ever need any of that stuff. Support groups are great for people that really need to know there are other people out there like them so they don't feel isolated and so much a failure. But I don't feel that way. If we don't have kids, I don't think I'll ever consider myself a failure as the result of it, even if it were diagnosed as my problem." Although Lee had been diagnosed as having a reproductive impairment, he still did not feel a strong need for support: "I could probably deal with infertility fairly well without Resolve. I don't think my wife could. I think maybe I've got a little bit out of it, but without it I probably wouldn't be a basket case. I could probably deal pretty well with my feelings and with our infertility, I think."

Although husbands claim not to need support, something else may be operating here as well. As we have seen in Chapter 5, men are less inclined than women to expressiveness and self-disclosure. Husbands may not feel as much of a *need* for support as their wives, but they may also feel less comfortable *asking* for support. It should be remembered, too, that "support" in support groups often means supportive talk. Husbands might be more comfortable with forms of support, such as giving concrete help to others, that are more in accordance with male modes of expressing intimacy.

Wives who wanted the benefits of a support group but whose husbands weren't interested responded in different ways. Carol felt that she could profit from involvement with a support group, but she stayed away because Stuart wasn't willing to go to meetings:

> Stuart's never had a desire to do that. At the time, I never felt like I had a good argument to discuss it. We discussed it, of course, and he came up with a simple reason, "Well, why do I want to sit around with all these people crying about something, when I know how I feel?" And, at the time, I guess maybe I was too overwhelmed with the idea of it's not happening, I don't know. All I know is I never had a really good argument to make him decide that maybe this is what we should do.

Because Lee wasn't interested in going to Resolve meetings with her, Robin decided to go by herself:

> I'm really shy of going into new groups of people all by myself. And so I needed the support of him to go with me, and he wasn't always available to go with me because socializing with infertile people wasn't on his top of his priority list, I don't think. His golf and his tennis were. And so we didn't make it to things all that often, but after a while, I got myself going.

Even the husbands who did attend Resolve meetings tended to get less involved in Resolve activities than their wives. Tom described an unsuccessful attempt to organize special activities for men:

> Resolve seems to revolve around more of the women's point of view. Women seem to want that more than the guys. Once a month is a women's coffee. Just the women get together at

somebody's house. There was an attempt there for a while to have a men's coffee, and that just died abysmally. Nobody was interested in doing that. Guys get together and talk football. Nobody bares their feelings.

It is, of course, not surprising that wives experienced a greater need for support than their husbands. Nor is it surprising that wives were more likely to be active in Resolve. I have suggested that the root of the felt stigma of infertility is a powerful sense of failure occasioned by one's inability to act out a socially approved and personally accepted life script. Because feelings of failure are much stronger in wives than in their husbands, it is to be expected that wives would feel more isolated from the fertile world and that wives would experience more discomfort in their interactions with friends, acquaintances, and relatives. Thus, infertile wives are most likely to feel and act on the need for a new reference group capable of validating their feelings and restoring their sense of normalcy.

But even those husbands who do feel a need for support may still find it difficult to express their feelings in public. Chip discussed his reasons for not participating more actively in Resolve:

It's funny. I felt very uncomfortable. I enjoyed being at the meeting. I enjoyed the people, but I didn't want to contribute. I just kind of sat in the background. I liked being sort of the fly on the wall. It was great to hear people say the things that you were thinking. To me, that was tremendous. I mean that was great to think that they're going through the same thing, that the thoughts you're having are not unusual, that you're not a jerk for saying that or thinking that. But I really didn't feel comfortable enough to participate in sharing and standing up and saying, "Hey, listen to me, here's my thought."

Thus, there are probably two distinct reasons why husbands are less involved with support groups than their wives: not only may they feel less need for support, but they may also be less comfortable giving and accepting support.

It should be clear by now that the infertile, especially infertile wives, experience infertility as a major life crisis that shatters taken-for-granted assumptions about the course of their lives. Confronted by such crises, people often ask themselves, Why me? They struggle to make sense out of their experience.

SEVEN

WHY ME?
Infertility and the Search for Meaning

T he experience of infertility is an experience of biographical disruption.[1] Infertile people, especially infertile wives, experience infertility as an unexpected, unwelcome, and unpredictable hiatus in a life that had been proceeding according to a course that is both culturally prescribed and personally endorsed. For most infertile wives and some infertile husbands in my study, infertility spoiled both identity and interaction with the fertile world. For almost all the infertile couples I spoke with, infertility increased tension in their marriages and resulted in a less satisfactory sexual relationship.

When people experience such radical disruptions in their lives, they typically try to make sense out of what has happened to them. Human suffering calls out for explanation. When life goes awry, for ourselves or those closest to us, we discover ourselves wondering "why bad things happen to good people."[2] A well-known study of twenty-nine individuals who had been paralyzed in serious accidents found that all these accident victims had asked, Why me?[3] These individuals, then, saw their paralysis not only as a physical crisis but also as a crisis of meaning.

Why Me?

THE PROBLEM OF THEODICY

The task of providing meaning, of making sense out of chaotic and apparently meaningless experience, is an important social-psychological function that social scientists attribute to religion. All religious belief systems must work out solutions to the problem of theodicy—that is, the problem of providing humanly meaningful explanations for suffering, death, and other meaning-threatening situations.[4] For example, the Hindu tradition interprets suffering as retribution for wrong-doing in previous lives. Within the Judeo-Christian tradition, the most common explanations for suffering have centered around the notions of "God's will" and suffering as punishment for sin.

Therefore, any catastrophic health crisis necessarily presents itself to us in two guises. On the one hand, a health crisis is a technical problem: a malfunctioning body must be restored to health. On the other hand, a health crisis is an interpretive problem: a deviation from the expected and desired course of events must be explained in culturally meaningful terms.[5] In traditional societies, the technical and interpretive aspects of health problems are typically intertwined. The same individuals and institutions are responsible for both treating the individual and helping the individual make sense of his or her experience.

To illustrate this point, let me return to the Ndembu of Zambia, whose infertility rituals I described in Chapter 1. You may recall that the Ndembu believe that infertility results when a women is caught by the shade of a recently deceased maternal ancestor, presumably because she has not been devoting sufficient attention to her maternal kin. Ndembu infertility rituals seek to propitiate the afflicting shade by giving the deceased the attention she has been denied. The rituals, then, address simultaneously the technical problem of infertility and the problem of meaning; the rituals are directed simultaneously toward restoring fertility and explaining a woman's misfortune. Ndembu infertility beliefs perform another function. In Chapter 1, we saw that conflicting loyalties are endemic in this society where women live with their husbands' kin but are believed to owe primary allegiance to their own kin. In a society where the tension between women's loyalties to their own kin and to their husbands' kin are, so to speak, built into the social structure, the survival of the cultural emphasis on the matrilineal principle depends on the existence of some kind of sanction.

Like most traditional societies, the Ndembu offer women few alternatives to the roles of child-bearer and child-rearer. In such a society, to be without children is one of the greatest tragedies that can befall a woman. I would assert that, consciously or not, the Ndembu have come up with a sanction worthy of the importance of the matrilineal principle. The Ndembu association of infertility with violation of one's duties toward maternal kin helps enforce an important principle of Ndembu social structure by threatening the infliction of a dreadful punishment upon those who might be tempted to ignore it. Thus, the Ndembu explanation of infertility is both an interpretation of personal suffering and a mechanism of social control.

I suggest that all theodicies share this double aspect. Theodicies simultaneously explain suffering and warn people away from culturally proscribed behavior. In many societies, natural suffering is seized upon as an *occasion for social control*.[6] Because so many traditional societies place such high value on having children, many societies use the real threat of infertility to enforce behavioral norms that require the support of powerful sanctions. A belief that infertility is a result of promiscuity dampens tendencies to act promiscuously. Attributing infertility to quarrelsome behavior acts as a brake on quarrelsome behavior.

As a result of the Janus-faced character of theodicy, cultural explanations of suffering tend to "blame the victim." The Ndembu belief—infertility is due to a failure to be sufficiently loyal to one's matrilineal kin—implies that an infertile woman is personally responsible for her own affliction. People throughout the world blame the victim by attributing infertility to careless or evil-intentioned behavior on the part of the infertile themselves. Ethnographer V. Ebin studied twenty-five cases of female infertility treated by spirit mediums among the Aowin people of southwest Ghana and discovered that, in twenty-one out of the twenty-five cases, the spirit medium found that the woman had brought about her own plight, either by failing to properly observe ritual requirements or by quarreling with kin.[7] The infertile, of course, are not the only sufferers who find themselves blamed for their own misfortune. In all world cultures, people are stigmatized for possessing any number of undesirable traits or conditions.

This tendency of theodicies to blame the victim for his or her own suffering may mean that all theodicies have some built-in limitations to their ability to comfort sufferers. There may be comfort in having an explanation—any explanation—for one's unfortunate circumstances, but I assume individuals would find even greater comfort if culturally available interpretations did not hold them personally responsible for the misfortune that has befallen them. Thus, inherent in the very nature of theodicy is a contradiction between the goal of comforting sufferers and the need to hold individuals responsible for their own behavior.

Max Weber, the German sociologist who introduced the notion of theodicy to the sociology of religion, pointed out that there are "theodicies of good fortune" as well as theodicies of suffering.[8] To state Weber's point simply, theodicies can not only explain their suffering to sufferers, but also justify their good fortune to the relatively well off. I assert that *all* theodicies simultaneously endorse both suffering and good fortune. All culturally standardized explanations of human suffering attempt to account for both hardship and well-being. For example, the Ndembu belief that infertility punishes disloyalty to matrilineal kin implies that the fertile have been rewarded with children because they have observed cultural rules concerning proper behavior toward matrilineal kin. Because theodicies must attempt to show that virtue is rewarded and that the rewarded are virtuous, they also tend to hold that those who suffer deserve to suffer. Thus, although health practices and beliefs in traditional societies make suffering humanly meaningful, they often do this in a way that stigmatizes sufferers.

THE MEDICAL MODEL AND THE MEANING
OF HEALTH PROBLEMS

In contemporary American society, the treatment of health problems is dominated by the medical model, which locates the source of health problems within the human body.[9] Although traditional healing systems do not distinguish clearly between the technical and the interpretive aspects of health problems, the medical model draws a clear line between these two areas of concern and considers its sphere limited to technical issues. Furthermore, the medical model assumes that, once an organic problem has been identified, the health problem in question has been *fully accounted for*.[10] Not only does the medical model declare the interpretive and the technological aspect of health problems intellectually separable, but it also sees the interpretive aspect as irrelevant to its essentially technological mission.

The acceptance of the medical model represents the *secularization* of beliefs and practices regarding health. By secularization, I refer to the decline in the number of spheres of everyday life in which discourse about the sacred and questions about the ultimately significant are held appropriate. For example, in traditional societies, work is imbued with sacred significance. People regulate planting and other productive activities according to a sacred calendar. They often resort to supernatural sanctions to protect their land from theft. The rise of large-scale industrial and agricultural enterprises in the modern era has meant that work has become increasingly organized according to rational considerations. In the process, work has lost much of its former sacred significance. Workers in large-scale industrial enterprises neither look for nor find the same kind of sacred significance in production schedules that peasants in traditional agricultural societies often find in the cycle of the seasons. While peoples throughout the world have addressed the supernatural in attempts to assure their good harvests, few would consider taking the same kinds of action to insure the production of an excellent car.

Just as the rise of industrial bureaucracy represents the secularization of production in modern society, so does the rise of scientific medicine represent the secularization of health care. Questions of meaning and interpretation no longer hold a place in the science of medicine; they are relegated to religious institutions, medical ethicists, and individuals themselves who must work them out on their own. But the problem of theodicy does not go away. People who confront serious health crises continue to look for some ultimate meaning in what has befallen them.[11] They continue to ask, Why me?

Although people continue to pursue interpretation, the secularization represented by the dominant medical model may make it more difficult to find meaning in health crises by eroding the plausibility of nontechnical interpretations. In their study of parents of children with childhood leukemia, medical sociologists Jean Comoroff and Peter Maguire suggest that medical interpretations of health and illness may make it more difficult to impose meaning on the situation. A study of a community's response to a mine disaster found that residents saw religion as irrelevant to their plight because they attributed the disaster to human agency and technology rather than to divine or natural causes.[12]

Even though the medical model is an explicitly secular system of ideas, it still has an implicit theodicy.[13] Any world view has implications for the question of the nature of suffering. Implicit in the medical model's radical separation of the technical realm from the interpretive realm is the notion that suffering is *pointless*. Unlike traditional theodicies, the medical model's secular theodicy refuses to contemplate the meaning of suffering. This refusal to entertain questions of the meaning and interpretation of suffering implies that such questions are not worth thinking about.

And if the medical model has an implicit theodicy, then it also has an implicit moral imperative, an implicit prescription for action. If suffering is pointless, then it is pointless to suffer. The medical model's focus on the technical side of health problems implies that suffering is not something to be endured stoically but rather something to be cónquered by using all available technical resources. Suffering is viewed not as something to be explained but as something to be relieved.

Because the theodicy of technology implicit in the medical model denies that suffering has meaning, it would appear at first glance to avoid the tendency of most traditional theodicies to blame the victim. After all, according to the medical model, the cause of a malady is to be found only within the individual's body. But, more and more, medical thinking is embracing the idea that the individual is ultimately responsible for his or her own health.[14] This notion, when combined with the insistence that all health problems have technical explanations, leads naturally to the idea that the source of health problems is individuals' failure to properly monitor and maintain their body-machines. For example, now that heart attacks have been linked to diet, the opportunity is ripe for developing the idea that heart attack victims have brought about their own plight by failing to maintain a proper diet. Even where the link between behavior and body is less clear, the suspicion may remain that people are ultimately responsible for the failures of their own bodies.

Thus, secular theodicies may be just as prone to blame the victim as traditional theodicies. We have already seen that the infertile, especially infertile wives, have a strong tendency to see their infertility as personal failure; and this pervasive sense of failure overshadows their relationships with representatives of the fertile world. From the victim's point of view, however, the medical model's implicit denial that suffering is humanly meaningful may be even more painful than the suggestion that individuals are ultimately responsible for what has befallen them.

A number of the infertile couples I interviewed embraced the pursuit of medical/technical solutions as the most plausible approach to dealing with the problem of infertility. How does their acceptance of the medical model affect these couples' ability to find meaning in the biographical disruption they confront? In this chapter, I examine the couples' attempts to make sense of the experience of infertility.

THEODICIES OF INFERTILE COUPLES

To elicit accounts from my respondents about how they had been affected by infertility at the level of meaning, I asked everyone, toward the end of the interview, "Did you ever ask yourself, 'Why is this happening to me?'" If respondents did not spontaneously offer a religious interpretation of infertility, then I asked directly if they had ever interpreted their infertility in religious terms.

I used two separate methods to estimate levels of religiosity among the couples in my sample. First, I examined transcripts for evidence of attendance at religious services and discovered that eleven wives and nine husbands mentioned habitual attendance at religious services. Second, I examined transcripts for spontaneous references to God or other language indicating belief in a transcendent reality. I found that nineteen wives and twelve husbands spontaneously used transcendent language during the course of their interviews.

Of the twenty-two couples in my sample, eighteen wives and eleven husbands described themselves as having asked the question, Why me? Of these, seventeen wives and eight husbands spontaneously used language that indicated their concern with God or a superempirical entity. I described these people as addressing this issue in a religious idiom. Jean is representative of those who posed the question, Why me? in a religious idiom: "We're not a very religious family. We go to church; we're Protestants. We were both brought up in church. But it was like, if there is this God who's this wonderful person, why is he doing this to us? We've been good people, we've played by the rules, and we've done what we should have done all of our lives. 'Why is he punishing us?' was how I felt." Stuart also employed a religious idiom in posing the question, Why me?:

> I am a very religious person, but it makes me angry when I read about people that kill their children, abuse their children, stuff them in garbage cans, or burn them. And I say to myself, "Why do you give children to these people and others and not to

me?" You know, "What the hell did I do wrong?" I know I didn't do anything wrong. I still don't understand it today.

Some of those who addressed the issue in religious terms, usually wives, reported being angry with God. Kate said she felt this way: "Well, I usually direct my anger at God, and when I'm angry, I'd say I'm angry at Him. I'm just sort of angry at the way life has turned out, you know. I guess I have not really accepted it." Janet, who took her Catholicism very seriously, stopped going to church to get back at God for what He had done to her: "There's nobody I can really be bitter at other than God. It's terrible to say, but I've quit going to Mass because [voice faltering] I feel that God's let me down, that He's punishing me, and I've never done anything to deserve it."

Some wives I talked with reported going through a stage of bargaining with God. Cathy said that she went through such a stage: "I spent a few months working to get God on my side. I did the novenas, and I prayed for lengthy periods of time at night, before I went to bed. I made little bargains, like, 'If you let me get pregnant this month, I promise this.' I found myself doing that sort of thing for a period of time and then decided, well, that's not the answer."

Not everyone who asked, Why me? posed the question in a religious idiom. One wife and three husbands asked the question without resorting to transcendent language. The following excerpt from my conversation with Dan provides an example of the secularized Why me? question:

Interviewer: Have you ever asked yourself, Why me?
Dan: Yeah. Probably about an hour ago when I was driving home. I do that all the time. Kind of one of those rhetorical questions. Philosophical things.
Interviewer: Have you come up with answers?
Dan: Absolutely not.

Dan's wife Sherry also asked Why me? without making use of transcendent language:

Interviewer: Did you ever ask, Why me, why is this happening to me?

Sherry: Yeah, a lot.

Interviewer: How did you answer yourself?

Sherry: I didn't come up with an answer. I just decided that life is unfair, and that probably wasn't a good answer. I always thought I was a good person. I always tried to do good things for people. I just decided that it just really wasn't fair. It used to really gall me when somebody would get pregnant the first month they would try to get pregnant without even trying. It seems so unfair.

Sherry reported that she too had gone through a bargaining stage, although she was not specific about who or what she was bargaining with: "I guess I went through that bargaining stage where you say, 'If you just let me have a baby, I'll go to church for the next fifty years.'"

I find it interesting that, even though Sherry avoided using the term God or any other language that suggested she believed in a personal, transcendent deity, she still felt the temptation to bargain, to address the "something" she believed in as if it were a person. She seems to me to be caught between two worlds. On the one hand, it seems she has a secular world view. Life, she says, is just unfair. But, on the other hand, she does not quite seem comfortable with the notion that there is no reason for her suffering. Sherry seems to think that life *ought* to be fair, that it ought to make sense. She seems unwilling to let go entirely of the notion that something "out there" might be propitiated. The remaining four wives and eleven husbands denied thinking much about the meaning of infertility. An excerpt from the transcript of an interview with Matt illustrates this point of view:

Interviewer: Did you ever, when you were going through this, sit back and ask yourself, "Why me?"

Matt: Nope. No, I didn't feel like God was giving me a ration of crap or anything like that.

Of those who denied giving much thought to the Why me? question, two wives and two husbands attributed infertility to chance or fate. When I asked Carol "Did you ever ask yourself, why me?" she answered: "Maybe it's fatalism. I just think that everybody has things that are wrong. Everybody has problems, and this has been mine. And why me instead of somebody else? Why should I be lucky enough to have a nice house when somebody else doesn't? You know, that's what I got, and that's nice. And being able to have a baby is what I didn't get, and that's too bad. And I don't know." Lee saw infertility as "just one of those things that happen": "Occasionally I've wondered about it, but I never really delve into it too much. It's just one of those things that happen. I don't think it's because I did this or that when I was younger or because I'm being punished for something."

It should be clear by now that, while both husbands and wives asked the Why me? question, wives were more likely both to pose it and to pose it in a sacred idiom. Husbands were more likely to take infertility in their cognitive stride. This may be partly owing to the greater religiosity of women in American society. It is probably also, at least partly, owing to the fact that the sense of identity and self-esteem of wives rather than of husbands is more likely to be threatened by infertility (see Chapter 3). Because wives are most likely to experience infertility in terms of failure, it is not at all surprising that wives rather than their husbands are more likely to find previous constructions of reality threatened and to experience infertility not only as a health problem but also as a cognitive crisis. Finally, because wives are expected to be the emotional specialists in marriage, developing accounts of emotionally charged experiences may be regarded by both wives and husbands as part of "women's work."[15]

SEARCHING FOR ANSWERS

Many people I spoke with asked, Why me? But few came up with convincing answers. Of the seventeen wives and eleven husbands who reported asking, Why me? only two wives and three husbands seem to have settled on answers with which they were satisfied. Two wives and one husband saw their infertility as God's will. Here is how Peg put it:

> I'm not super religious, but I just felt that if this is what God wanted, He has His reasons for everything. The same with death. You know, you could be sitting here on this couch, or you could have a car accident. If you're going to die, you're going to die; it doesn't matter where you are or what you're doing. And I guess I just figured maybe God just had something else in mind for us. Cliff and I talked about it. Maybe we are supposed to help other people with children in some way.

My sample includes two husbands who saw infertility as a sort of punishment. Dave felt that God was withholding a child from his wife Martha because she wasn't emotionally ready to have a child. Roger thought that the stillbirth of his son might have been a punishment for his getting angry at his wife Kate. However, the vast majority of those who ask, Why me? are unable to come up with satisfying answers. Janet is typical of this group:

> *Interviewer:* Do you ever ask yourself, why me?
> *Janet:* Uh huh. Many times.
> *Interviewer:* And what do you answer?
> *Janet:* [nervous laugh] I don't know.
> *Interviewer:* I mean, do you ever think about it in religious terms?
> *Janet:* Why God's punishing me? Uh huh [nervous laugh].
> *Interviewer:* But you really haven't come up with any explanation for why it's happening to you that satisfies you?
> *Janet:* No, no.

Among those I consider unable to answer, Why me? I discern two groups: those who think, as Brett does, that "there must be a reason" but aren't sure what it is; and those who suspect this may be punishment but don't know what for. Robin mused about some thoughts that go through her mind when she asks herself, Why me?:

> I must have done something wrong when I was a little kid. And I was always stupid. Uh, let's see. . . . Oh, God always took away everything I loved, so of course He wouldn't let me have children. That was usually it. I saw myself as the type of person that everything always went wrong for, so why would this go right? I was just following the characteristics of my life.

Debby toyed with the idea that her infertility was a punishment for actions in the past. Although she ultimately rejected this line of thought, she still felt guilty:

> Being Catholic I think has something to do with it. When I was younger and was involved with someone before I was married and thought I was pregnant, I remember thinking, "If I am not pregnant now, I'll trade this for getting pregnant ten years from now when I want to be." And I'm thinking that somehow this magical thinking could have caused that. Well, of course it didn't, but I still feel guilty that I traded my soul to the devil.

Karen tearfully expressed her inability to explain what has happened to her. Although she came up with an answer, the text suggests that she was not sure she put much stock in it:

> I don't really blame God, but sometimes I wonder. God knows how much I love children. I just can't figure out why He doesn't let me have some. I mean, I believe very strongly He can do whatever He wants. And some people say that maybe there's a reason, and other people say that "Well, God doesn't really actively intervene in our lives." So maybe there's a child overseas that just absolutely really needs us, and this is the only way He could make that come out. That's the only thing I can think of.

People like Robin, Debby, and Karen are puzzled by their infertility. They think there must be some reason for their suffering, and they call upon their religious backgrounds in their attempts to develop convincing interpretations. But they seem unable to answer, Why me? to their own satisfaction. They experiment with possible answers, but they put these answers forward tentatively, almost apologetic that these are the best they have.

I am struck by the number of people who considered but then rejected the possibility that infertility was a punishment for a past misdeed. Jean asked, "Why is He punishing us?" Stuart wondered, "What the hell did I do wrong?" Janet complained that she was being punished without doing anything to deserve it. To people like Jean and Stuart and Janet, infertility definitely *feels* like a punishment, and they are certainly familiar with the cultural notion that suffering is a punishment for sin. That so many people refer to the notion of suffering as punishment indicates that this idea still has a powerful appeal in our culture. Yet, they do not appear to have seriously undertaken a spiritual quest to explain their infertility. Rather, they seem to reject out of hand the idea that they might actually *deserve* to be punished. Although the notion of suffering as punishment is pervasive, it seems to have lost some plausibility. Most people I spoke to raised the issue of infertility as punishment only to make the point that this could not possibly be the reason for their suffering. People are aware of the explanations of suffering offered by traditional theodicies, but they do not seem comfortable using them as resources to be drawn upon in their attempt to find meaning in their situation.

Not only was it difficult to employ religious resources to make sense of infertility, but some people found that the experience of infertility threatened the validity of previous constructions of reality. This excerpt is from my interview with Jean, who had a three-year-old adopted son at the time of the interview:

Interviewer: Did it shake your faith?
Jean: Oh yeah.

Interviewer: Do you think that you became less religious because of it?
Jean: Yeah, I would say so.
Interviewer: Have you become more religious now?
Jean: No.

It seems to me that the crucial distinction to be drawn here is between those who either found an answer to Why me? or didn't ask the question, on the one hand, and those who continued to find the question troubling, on the other. I describe the latter group as finding infertility threatening at the level of meaning and the former group as not finding it so. By dividing the respondents this way, we find that fifteen wives and eight husbands found infertility threatening at the level of meaning while seven wives and fourteen husbands did not. Thus, it would be hard to argue that the individuals in this sample found religious theodicies an important source of meaning upon which they could draw in their attempt to deal with the crises of infertility.

Because religion is often credited as an important resource for the construction of meaning, one might expect that the more religious people in my sample would be less likely to find infertility threaten the level of meaning. But this does not appear to be the case. Rather, both husbands and wives who used transcendent language spontaneously seemed *more* likely to find infertility a threat to meaning than those who did not; likewise, both wives and husbands who reported attending religious services regularly were more likely to see infertility as a threat to meaning than those who did not. [16]

Thus religion does not provide meaning for my respondents, as one might expect; religion does not provide most couples in my sample with resources upon which they can call to explain to themselves their experience of suffering. The majority of those in my sample who reported seeking meaning in the experience of infertility seemed dissatisfied with the progress of their search.

One might expect that individuals with documented reproductive impairments would be more likely than those whose spouses who have documented reproductive impairments to find infertility threatening to meaning. This does not seem to be the case for the wives in my sample—not particularly surprising, given that wives experience the impact of infertility upon their identities whether they have a documented reproductive impairment or not. Husbands, however, are somewhat more likely to see infertility as a threat to meaning when the problem is biologically "their own." This is not surprising either, given the fact that the impact of infertility on identity is greater for husbands who themselves have a diagnosed reproductive impairment than among those who do not.[17]

Not only do many people I interviewed find it difficult to accept their infertility and deal with it religiously, but some interpret others' attempts to help them accept their infertility as evidence that the others do not understand the infertility experience. Two excerpts from interviews with wives illustrate this point. Debby saw her mother's belief that her infertility was God's will as an obstacle to overcome:

Interviewer: Is your mother pretty supportive?
Debby: In her own way. She tends to be pretty religious and accepted things that I would have been really pissed off about. You know, "It's God's will" kind of stuff. I made a comment to her; I said I was going out with a friend who had adopted a Korean kid. I said "because I'm getting nervous about ever being able to conceive and I just need to talk about adoption." And she said, "It will all work out." And I think she believes that.

Sherry saw her parents' admonishments that she should accept her infertility and move on with her life as evidence that they were less supportive than they ought to have been: "My parents—it's been absolutely amazing to me—they have not been supportive. They don't understand why we are making this into a big deal and can't accept what's happened. You know, 'That's the way it is, so move on with it.'"

By the time I interviewed them, twelve couples had been successful in their quest to become parents, by either having a biological child or adopting one. Some people who now have children are able to look at the experience of infertility retrospectively and see a pattern to what once appeared as chaos. Liz, whose two-year-old adopted son Ryan was in the room with us during our interview, related: "I don't think I could have accepted infertility without having some positive resolution come out of it and still have faith because I was getting quite upset. But because things did work out, I have much more faith. I just really feel that God played a big part in it all. All the way around, I have much more faith."

Cathy became pregnant shortly after adopting a child. During our interview, she talked about the meaning she has found in her good fortune: "I don't find myself attending church more, but I find myself thanking God constantly. I wake up in the morning, and I take a look at my son and I say, 'Thank you for this beautiful little boy.' I feel the baby move inside me, and I say, 'Thank you for letting me have this experience.' I talk to God a lot more." For Liz, Cathy, and others like them, a religious solution to the problem of meaning came only after there was a child in the home. Thus, for many, infertility appeared a threat to meaning, a catastrophe that could not easily be assimilated into existing constructions of reality as long as they remained childless. Only after these wives had dealt with infertility *practically* were they able to deal with it abstractly. The theodicies they constructed, then, were not theodicies of suffering but theodicies of good fortune.

Many people in my sample found it difficult to bring religious resources to bear in their attempt to make sense of the experience of infertility. Some people still found some satisfaction in their involvement with religious institutions. There is, after all, a kind of meaning in belonging, too. Some of the same people who were unable to construct satisfying religious interpretations of infertility still found the social support they received in church rewarding and meaningful. An excerpt from my interview with Jean illustrates this point:

Jean: Well, we've had a good relationship with our church mainly to help us with adoption. Because our adoption agency is very religiously oriented. We needed a clergy reference and this and that, so we've been really good about going to church for the last three years or so.

Interviewer: So your reaction religiously is that you're pleased with the institution, but you're not sure your faith is where it was before?

Jean: Right. I enjoy church as far as the social end of it. We have friends at church; the music is lovely; we have a wonderful choir. But no, I don't think my faith is where it was before, no.

Stuart also commented on the social rewards of church attendance: "Without getting religious or anything, the people have been so nice and just like a big family."

Those who talked about religious institutions as supportive and helpful, however, were far outnumbered by those who talked about a religious organization as one more obstacle to be overcome in their struggle to cope with infertility (see Chapter 3).

EXPLAINING THE FAILURE OF THEODICY

What are we to make of the fact that many infertile people are trying but, for the most part, failing to make religious sense of infertility? We must consider the possibility that my results are at least partly an artifact of my sampling technique. Because most couples I interviewed are either members of Resolve or part of social networks that involve Resolve members, I may have oversampled individuals who are particularly treatment-oriented. Such individuals might be less likely than others to be able to find meaning in their situation. In fact, their inability to deal cognitively with infertility may be one factor that leads such people to seek out support groups like Resolve. As it happens, the Resolve members in my sample were more likely than non-Resolve members to find infertility a threat to meaning.[18] Thus, we cannot rule out the possibility that the couples we interviewed may be less able or willing to deal with infertility at the level of meaning than other couples. Still, comparing other studies of the search for meaning with these situations of suffering suggests that difficulties in constructing satisfying theodicies are not unique to this sample. There are several plausible conclusions to draw from my discussion.

First, theodicies may just not work all that well. The need for theodicy exists, after all, because threats to meaning are plentiful. Perhaps religious attempts to explain suffering are doomed always to be, at best, only partially successful. It is perhaps telling that none of the few social scientific studies of meaning construction in situations of suffering provides convincing evidence that people are able to build theodicies that provide them with meaning and comfort. One study of forty-one individuals whose spouses had died in automobile accidents and thirty-nine individuals who had lost children under similar circumstances found that 69 percent of those who had lost spouses and 59 percent of those who had lost children reported that they were unable to find meaning in their loss. Of the spouses, 85 percent had asked themselves, Why me? The figure for parents was 91 percent. In both groups, 59 percent of the respondents reported finding no satisfactory answer to the Why me? question. In a study of parents of children with childhood leukemia, medical sociologists Jean Comaroff and Peter Maguire discovered that few parents found religious explanations viable.[19]

Moreover, theodicies of good fortune may be inherently more stable than theodicies of suffering. The people I spoke to had a much easier time making sense of infertility after they had adopted a child or given birth to a child. The tendency of theodicies of suffering to blame victims for their own misfortune may limit their usefulness as resources for building meaning. Many people I spoke to were unwilling to entertain seriously the notion that their infertility was a punishment for something they had done wrong. Similarly, only two of the twenty-nine accident victims studied by social psychologists Ronnie Bulman and Camille Wortman felt that their paralyzing accidents were deserved.[20]

Second, I focus my concern on the chronic nature of infertility.

Couples experience infertility as a chronic crisis, something that permeates every aspect of their lives, something that simply will not go away. Some evidence suggests that people may be more successful in finding meaning in acute crises than in chronic crises. An examination of the studies we have reviewed suggests that people may be more successful in constructing theodicies to deal with death than they are in constructing theodicies to deal with illness. Studies of patients experiencing chronic pain suggest that chronic suffering is particularly resistant to attempts to construct meaning.[21]

The study of the spouses and the parents of accident victims discussed earlier in this section found that people experienced loss of spouse as more of a threat to meaning than the loss of a child. The authors speculate that this is because a spouse is an important source of support, but it might also stem from the fact that people's everyday experiences and daily routines are more likely to be affected by the loss of a spouse than by the loss of a child (unless the child was an only child).[22] Insofar as infertility is experienced as a master status that permeates much of everyday life, we might expect that it, too, is particularly resistant to attempts at constructing meaning.

Third, the open-ended nature of infertility challenges theodicy building. Comaroff and Maguire found that uncertain prognoses made it particularly difficult for parents of children with leukemia to make sense out of their situation.[23] As we have seen, infertile couples do not see parenthood as something denied them once and for all; rather, they see themselves as not yet pregnant. The open-endedness of infertility makes it difficult for the members of an infertile couple to say, "Oh well, I guess it's just God's will," and get on with their lives.

Finally, as our understanding of reproduction has been medicalized, reproduction has lost some aura of the mysterious and the miraculous that it once had. Reproduction is no longer understood as something that "just happens" but rather as a biological process that humans can hope to master. Infertility appears not as a mysterious and unexplainable disability to be accepted but as a technical problem to be overcome. In such circumstances, traditional theodicies, which counsel stoicism in the face of the inevitable, may lose ground to the impatient theodicy implied by the medical model. According to the medical model, suffering is not something to be understood but rather something to be conquered. Explanations that rely on such concepts as "God's will" cannot be convincing when we believe as strongly as we do in the human ability to pull ourselves out of our condition through technical knowledge. To accept the kinds of answers traditional theodicies can give implies a spirit of resignation. Such a spirit of resignation does not currently exist in the pursuit of infertility treatment.

The same developments that have made infertility easier to handle practically may have made it harder to handle cognitively. The development of reproductive technology, like other medical advances, presents us with a paradox. As our ability to deal with health problems in technical terms increases, our ability to deal with them at the level of meaning may decrease.

EIGHT

CONCLUSIONS
Infertility, Present and Future

We have been listening to the wives and husbands of twenty-two infertile couples describe for us their encounter with infertility—how they felt about it, and how it has affected them. Perhaps it makes sense at this juncture to systematically summarize some key features of the contemporary experience of infertility.

INFERTILITY IN A CONTEMPORARY CONTEXT

First, we can safely generalize that infertility was experienced differently by wives and husbands. For most wives, infertility brought with it a deeply felt sense of personal failure. Infertility posed a devastating threat to identity; it was a problem they thought about often and one they could not easily escape. Wives often immersed themselves in the task of solving their infertility problems, actively seeking treatment and reading voraciously on the subject. Husbands, especially those without reproductive impairments, were more likely to regard infertility as an unfortunate circumstance, but as one that could be put into perspective and handled accordingly. For many husbands, the main problem with infertility was that their wives were unhappy and that home life had become less enjoyable than it had once been.

174

For many couples, these gender-based differences in the experience of infertility produced frustration and tension within the marital relationship. Wives sometimes saw their husbands as callous and unaffected by infertility, while husbands sometimes saw their wives as overreacting and obsessed. Although wives sometimes felt their husbands were unwilling to talk about infertility, some husbands wondered what there was to talk about.

Tension, frustration, and struggles over communication are by no means unique to infertile couples. (In fact, I have presented some evidence suggesting that, in the long run, infertility may have a salutary effect on a couple's level of communication.) That wives and husbands experience infertility differently is just one reflection of the fact that American wives and husbands live in different experiential worlds. American women and men have been and still are subject to different sets of expectations regarding attitudes, emotions, demeanor, and behavior. The new norms promoting the communicative marriage as the ideal thus require two people who have learned to experience the world in quite distinct ways to share one reality, or at least to act as if they do. Just as other American couples do, infertile couples find the attempt to share their experience a challenging task. And, just as other American couples do, infertile wives and husbands often blame each other when they fall short of the ideal.

Second, central to the experience of the infertile, especially for infertile wives, is their strong awareness of the inability to conform to social norms that they themselves accept as valid. Infertility is thus associated with a sense that one has lost control over the ability to live according to one's life plan. It is experienced, not solely as a physical challenge, but also as an obstacle to making sense of one's own life.

Under such circumstances, apparently innocuous events of everyday life become for the infertile painful reminders of their sense of failure. Television commercials, chance encounters with passersby, conversations at work, insensitive comments by friends and relatives—all dramatize for the infertile, especially for infertile wives, their involuntary exile from normality. For the infertile wives and some infertile husbands I interviewed, infertility was experienced as a secret stigma, capable of spoiling interaction even when hidden from the view of others. Thus, many people I spoke with harbored a deep sense of loneliness, a feeling that their suffering was unrecognized and unappreciated by others. Because they felt that only those who shared their experience were really equipped to understand, many infertile wives and some infertile husbands turned to infertile friends and self-help groups for support.

The infertile are not alone in believing that only those who share their experience can provide them with a supportive community. Alcoholics, people with weight problems, and the chronically ill—just to name a few—all feel a need to construct communities of sufferers like themselves. Nor is the American tendency to seek out groups of others with similar characteristics limited to those with problems that have been defined as medical. Many Americans—Born-Again Christians, Moonies, environmentalists—are constructing new, ad hoc communities made up of people with perspectives similar to their own. Presumably, this is occurring because other institutions, such as family and workplace, are not satisfying important needs for support, understanding, and community. Perhaps this trend also indicates that many Americans feel they lack control of certain aspects of their lives and are actively trying to restore a sense of control.

Third, contemporary infertility has become defined by the medical profession, the general public, and infertile couples alike as a medical problem. As we have seen, infertility is in the process of becoming increasingly medicalized and industrialized. The infertile see medical institutions as able to solve their problems, and medical professionals are now more ready than ever before to proffer possible solutions.

But the solutions offered by most of the medical profession address only one small part of the problem of infertility. Guided by the medical model, doctors attend to the technical aspects of infertility and usually ignore social, emotional, and cognitive aspects. Furthermore, most infertility specialists concentrate on achieving the primary goal of a pregnancy and look to such nonmedical solutions for infertility as adoption and remaining childless only when attempts to achieve a pregnancy have proven futile.[1] Concerns about feelings of loneliness, about perceptions of failure, and about threats to the sense that the world is a meaningful place are sometimes acknowledged but rarely addressed.

The wives and husbands I interviewed accepted the correctness of the medical view of their problems as technical and controllable. They were often shocked and demoralized when they realized that birth isn't quite as controllable as they might once have thought, but they remained committed to technical solutions to what they perceived as medical problems. At the same time that they accept the validity of the medical model, however, infertile couples criticize medical institutions for not meeting their other needs. Left to their own resources, they rely on ad hoc devices like support groups and informal friendship networks to meet needs not being met elsewhere.

Here, too, we see that the infertile are a lot like other Americans. As more and more aspects of American life have become medicalized, we have come to rely increasingly on medical experts to solve our problems. But, at the same time, we have become more critical of the medical profession for its failure to live up to its promise. The medicalization of American society and the medical profession's loss of legitimacy are two sides of the same coin. What can be said about medicine can also be said about technology in general. Our faith in the ideology of technology is expanding: We have become increasingly intoxicated by the idea that every problem has a technical solution. But as we have become more committed to the ideology of technology, we have simultaneously become more disillusioned by technology's failure to live up to our expectations. And we have grown more aware that technology is incapable of addressing some types of problems—problems of meaning, for example. Still we remain committed to the search for technical solutions.

Fourth, because of the uncertain prognosis for most couples, infertility is experienced as a liminal state, a condition that the infertile can neither escape nor accept as inescapable. Many infertile couples harbor a realistic expectation for a medical solution, and nontreatment-related pregnancies are always possible; therefore, the despair of infertility is entwined with the constant hope that "maybe next month will be the month." Most infertile see themselves, not as permanently childless, but as *not yet pregnant*. Hope, however, can be a burden as well as a blessing. The open-endedness of infertility contributes to the sense that one has lost control over the ability to live according to one's life plan.

People confronted with a sense of meaninglessness and lost control might be expected to respond with helplessness and resignation, but because these infertile couples were committed to technical solutions and saw the hope for a solution as realistic, their response instead was to pursue whatever lines of action seemed to them most likely to lead to a baby. From most wives in my sample one senses that they had an overriding goal: motherhood. Couples judged treatment options primarily in terms of whether they appeared to involve the most efficient and practical use of resources to reach the goal of parenthood. The nature of these couples' contacts with health care professionals may have helped move them from a commitment to getting a baby toward a more specific commitment to pursue treatment.

Because there is always something that can be done, responsibility for stopping treatment lies clearly in the couple's hands. In other words, they must take responsibility for "giving up." They must say at some point in the treatment process, "We are not willing to go through any more." Without a clear standard on which to base such a decision, most couples find it exceedingly difficult to stop pursuing biological parenthood. The fertility orientation of infertile wives is thus a rational response to their situation, given the social setting in which they experience infertility.

The contemporary experience of infertility, then, reflects certain key themes in American society in general. We expect people who live in different experiential worlds—men and women—to share intimately with one another. When they fail to meet this expectation, we blame the individuals rather than the institutions and historical circumstances that have made this ideal so hard to realize. We continue to have faith in science and technology as a solution to all sorts of problems at the same time that we criticize them for not meeting certain types of human needs. We struggle to make sense out of experience without confidence in overarching world views. We place an incredible burden of responsibility upon individuals and families to solve their own problems and absolve social structure from responsibility. Thus infertility serves as a kind of cultural window, which can help us sharpen our perception of contemporary American social institutions.

IMPROVING THE CARE OF INFERTILITY PATIENTS

In the previous chapters, we have heard infertile wives and husbands express frustration with certain aspects of their medical treatment. It is fairly obvious that certain steps could be taken to improve the medical care of infertile patients. For example, better communication and disclosure of information should be encouraged among physicians. But significant reform in the care of the infertile requires more than simply coaxing physicians to improve upon certain social skills.

Some problems reported by infertile couples could be eased by a couple-centered approach to infertility treatment. Treatment of men should be integrated with the treatment of women. The couple, not the individual patient, should be seen as the focus for medical care. For couple-centered treatment to have any impact, it must mean more than encouraging gynecologists to refer their patients' husbands to urologists; couple-centered treatment means rather the establishment of infertility clinics where male and female members of couples may be treated in the same facility from the beginning.

In all infertility treatment, the couple's welfare, not a medical cure, should be the goal. Those who care for the infertile must be aware that medical problems are only a small part of the crisis of infertility. It is crucial to attend to not only the medical needs of infertile couples but also their social, emotional, and cognitive needs.

Counseling should therefore be regarded as a routine part of all infertility treatment rather than an unusual phenomenon, thought necessary only in extreme cases of psychological distress.[2] Counselors should discuss all options, not just those that involve medical treatment, with each couple. And counselors should be aware of and help couples prepare for the strain they may experience as a result of husbands and wives' potentially different reactions to infertility.

Clearly most physicians are currently ill-equipped to deliver the kind of multifaceted care that the infertile require. The currently dominant care model—in which a physician has primary responsibility for the care of a patient and refers to counselors, social workers, and other specialists only when the physician deems this necessary—needs to give way to a model in which a *care team* attends to the full range of needs of the infertile. Because infertility is more than simply a medical problem, it is not self-evident that a physician should be in charge of this care team. For example, most infertile couples I spoke with felt that nurses were more sensitive to the full range of infertility issues than were doctors; therefore, we ought to at least consider the viability of a model in which a nurse or other helping professional coordinates the overall care of the infertile while physicians retain responsibility for the strictly medical aspects of infertility.

It also seems clear that none of these reforms will occur unless the infertile themselves and their potential allies—consumer's groups, women concerned with health issues, feminists, sufferers from other chronic medical complaints—are vocal in promoting their own interests.

Although these suggested changes in the delivery of health care services for the infertile would improve the quality of infertility care, they would probably not fundamentally alter the experience of infertility. If the experience of infertility is—to some extent, at any rate—conditioned by its social structural context, then fundamental changes would likely come only as a result of significant changes in social institutions. The question of effecting changes in institutions is the realm of social policy, and I must now briefly turn my attention to such questions.

INFERTILITY AND SOCIAL POLICY

Much public policy debate over infertility centers around the acceptability of the "new" reproductive technology.[3] Unlike such countries as Great Britain and Australia, the United States has no formal policy with regard to reproductive technology. Although the federal government does not support research into IVF or related techniques and although it provides scant support for any type of infertility research, it has done little if anything to constrain private development of these technologies.[4]

Supporters of developing reproductive technology often approach the issue from a perspective of individual rights.[5] They argue that the right to individual autonomy and the corollary right to make decisions regarding one's own body should be applied to those who wish to have a child just as much as to those who wish not to have a child. The creation of new methods for achieving parenthood, they assert, is beneficial because it increases the number of choices open to infertile couples who want to have a baby. Adherents of individual rights tend to include advocates for the infertile, representatives of the scientific and medical communities, and—more generally—those who embrace a liberal legal philosophy.

One example of the kind of federal legislation supported by such individuals is HR 2956, introduced in Congress in the summer of 1989 but never passed; the bill would have provided funding to promote research on birth control and infertility.[6] At the state level, advocates for the infertile have worked on behalf of legislation mandating that health insurance carriers cover a greater proportion of infertility expenses, especially those related to high-tech treatments.[7]

Opposition to the development of reproductive technology comes

181

primarily from two quite divergent sources. One group may be referred to as conservative or traditional.[8] Conservative opponents sometimes argue that the development of reproductive technology involves unwarranted human interference with the natural order. Like Jerry Falwell, they assert that "God's way is still the best way."[9] Other conservatives emphasize that the development of reproductive technology threatens traditional beliefs, values, and practices, especially those associated with the institution of the family. Some argue, for example, that using genetic material (e.g., sperm or eggs) from a third party violates the sanctity of marriage. Others argue that research on and manipulation of gametes, embryos, and fetuses violate the rights of the unborn and the unconceived.

The second major group that is suspicious of the growth of reproductive technology approaches the question from a feminist perspective.[10] Some feminists who object to the development of medical and legal means for circumventing infertility do so because they fear it will have harmful consequences for women. Feminist critics often argue that, far from multiplying the options open to women, the further escalation of intervention into procreation will actually result in limiting women's choices. Some argue that, in the context of a strong motherhood mandate, women really do not have the power to say "no" to reproductive technology.[11] Others argue that the very existence of reproductive options makes it difficult to opt not to try the available procedures.[12] And many warn that, in the future, some women may actually be forced to use these technologies in the service of men and other women.

Many feminists fear that a reproductive technology developed in the context of a society in which men have more power than women could not help but operate to the detriment of women. Many worry that the intervention into procreation signals a movement of control over birth and conception from the bodies of women to the hands of doctors, scientists, and the state and that women will thereby lose one of their most important sources of power and identity.[13] Some feminists argue that reproductive technology leads to a state of affairs in which women's reproductive capacities—and even children themselves—come to be regarded as commodities. [14] Andrea Dworkin, for example, has conjured up the image of a "reproductive brothel" in which women will sell their wombs, ovaries, and eggs for the use of others much as prostitutes sell their sexual capacities. [15] Many feminists fear the specter of a society in which people are "designed" in test tubes according to the principles of eugenics.

Another criticism launched by many feminists against reproductive technology is that it will benefit some women at the expense of others. Critics frequently note that only middle-class, mostly white women can afford to avail themselves of the new techniques for countering infertility; they point to the irony of helping privileged women have babies at the same time that sterilization and other forms of birth control are being foisted upon Third World women. Some look to a future in which poor women's reproductive capacities will be expropriated for the benefit of wealthy women.

How seriously should we take the objections put forward by traditionalists and feminists? I personally remain unconvinced by conservative arguments. The argument that reproductive technology involves illegitimate tampering with nature would, if taken to its logical extreme, entail the rejection of all types of medical intervention to treat infertility. The conservative rejection of intervention into procreation on the grounds that it threatens traditional values and practices sanctifies one possible social order as the only acceptable one and rejects out of hand the possibility of viable alternative social orders.

Furthermore, I do not think that the development of reproductive technology necessarily means the demise of the family. Far from seeing it as a threat to traditional family values, I think it more likely that reproductive technology will be employed to shore up traditional values. For example, most IVF clinics implant all fertilized eggs in the uterus to avoid criticism from Catholics and others who feel that allowing a fertilized egg to die is tantamount to abortion. Many IVF clinics limit their clientele to married couples.

Nor do I believe that the most horrifying predictions of some feminist writers will come to pass. I do not think the "reproductive brothel" is just around the corner. I am not convinced that IVF is going to become the required reproductive method for all couples. I don't think that the majority of American women are going to rush out and obtain the sperm of Nobel Prize winners in order to give birth to geniuses.

But the main concerns of the feminist critics may not be put aside so lightly. The data presented in this book support the claim that there is a coercive element to reproductive technology. The medicalization and industrialization of infertility is, perhaps, making it more difficult for the infertile, especially infertile women, to refrain from trying every possible alternative before giving up the quest for a biological child. My data also support the assertion that many women feel the normative pressure of the motherhood mandate so strongly that they do not feel free to choose not to pursue parenthood.

Evidence in my interviews also lends credence to the fear that the continued development of reproductive technology may give the medical profession greater control over women's bodies. In Chapter 4, I showed that the medical encounter is often the scene of a struggle between women and their doctors for control over the course of treatment. The escalating medicalization of reproduction during the course of the twentieth century has meant that women are increasingly living lives punctuated by medical intervention in ways that men's lives are not. The development of new methods of treating and circumventing infertility have contributed to both the increased medicalization of the lives of women and the loss of control that comes with medicalization.

Ironically, the increasing involvement of medical professionals in women's lives has contributed to both the general dissatisfaction many Americans feel with the medical profession and a stronger "consumer orientation" among patients. The declining legitimacy of medicine may, one hopes, ultimately lead to reforms that will return to patients a sense of greater control over their own bodies.

Proponents and opponents of reproductive technologies differ in their perception of both the dynamics of the rise of the new techniques and the infertile's role in that process. Supporters often argue that the development of reproductive technology is propelled by demand from infertile couples and that, because so many couples desperately want a child, it is proper to do anything reasonable to satisfy that wish. Opponents argue that people, especially women, are pressured into using the new reproductive technologies and are therefore more properly described as being exploited by these technologies than as taking advantage of them.

In my view, infertile women are neither the lucky beneficiaries of the new reproductive technology nor its hapless victims. Rather they have been active participants in bringing about a process that also exploits them. [16] Catherine Kohler Riessman has argued that the medicalization of women's lives has occurred when doctors' interests to maximize their professional power converges with the perceived medical needs of women, especially relatively affluent white women. [17] My data (see Chapter 2) support this interpretation. The growth of reproductive technologies is fueled by both middle-class couples' demands (such as those manifested among my interviewees) and physicians' professional interests.

How are we to balance the desires of infertile couples for treatment against the possible risks involved in the further development of reproductive technology? Should the infertile be called upon, as some feminist writers assert, to forgo treatment and sacrifice deeply desired goals for the sake of the long-range interests of women as a group? [18] Some arguments against reproductive technology seem to contain an element of blaming the victim. In effect, infertile couples are being told that they simply shouldn't place such a high value on parenthood. I think the preceding chapters have made it clear that the infertile are not likely to relinquish their claims to voluntary treatment voluntarily.

One great danger of the continued development of new reproductive technology is that it will split women apart, separating liberal feminists from radical feminists, dividing those who fear reproductive technology from those who wish to benefit from it, and turning those who can become pregnant against those who cannot. [19] Women united are more likely to prevent abuses of reproductive technology than are women divided. It is therefore in the interest of feminists to work toward a policy on reproductive technology that the infertile can live with. Alison Solomon has urged feminists to take up infertility as a feminist issue by establishing programs of "infertility crisis counseling."[20] I agree that much can be gained if feminists can find ways to attend to the infertile's concerns. The solution to the problem of reproductive technology is not to go back to the past, which is probably impossible anyway, but to determine how we can live with the present.

In contrast, some supporters of reproductive technology assume that any technological improvement will necessarily improve the quality of life of infertile couples and increase their range of choices. Any acceptable social policy must allow infertile couples the option of pursuing parenthood, but the best policy may not necessarily be the one that makes it easiest to generate the most technological breakthroughs, giving the infertile even more things to try.[21] We don't have a choice about whether to make social policy: Social policy will be made. If we do not make policy consciously then we will make it unconsciously through the decisions of courts, hospital administrators, and physicians. I would much rather see us consciously accept responsibility and decide how to use this technology.

As we attempt to forge a social policy, we must keep in mind that the problem is not primarily with the technology in and of itself but rather with the social context in which it is being created. Technology does not exist in a social vacuum. Not all of reproductive technology's consequences are inevitable by-products of its development. It is true, for example, that reproductive technology makes it easier for us to commodify reproduction by making it simpler for us to obtain eggs, sperm, and embryos to exchange, but the technology does not make us exchange them. It is also true that reproductive technology has been used primarily to benefit middle-class women while poor women are left to suffer with infertility, but, again nothing inherent in the technology requires this state of affairs. It is true that more effort is currently expended to circumvent infertility through developing reproductive technology than is spent trying to prevent infertility, but technology itself does not make medical institutions underemphasize prevention.

Reproductive technology is being developed in a specific social context. One important feature of that context is the existence of radical differences in the roles women and men are expected to play and in the degree to which they have access to power. It is because men have more power than women that feminists fear that men will control reproductive technology and use it to control women. Another relevant feature of the social context is an economy based on the production and exchange of commodities. Because we live in a society where many things—manufactured goods, songs, algorithms—are patented, marketed, and sold, it is not unreasonable to fear that sperm, eggs, and embryos could also be patented, marketed, and sold. American society is characterized by pervasive class and racial inequality, and it is for this reason that reproductive technology is employed for the benefit of some couples and not others.

American society has witnessed a trend toward the increasing power of the medical profession and an increasing role for medicine in social control, especially in the social control of women. Given past trends, it does not seem unreasonable to fear that the development of reproductive technology will result in an even greater involvement in social control for medicine. Most physicians are oriented toward somewhat narrowly focused cures for diseases rather than toward more broadly formulated notions of health. This fact helps explain why more energy is devoted to trying to "fix" infertility than to prevent it (for example, by reducing the incidence of pelvic inflammatory disease).

A strong historical tendency to genetic thinking has given rise to the idea that parenthood is biological and that adoptive parents and others who "merely" care for children are not "real" parents. This belief that parenthood is really a question of genes leads many to fear that the infertile would do *anything* to have a biological child. (We have seen, however, that many infertile couples I spoke with are more interested in having children than in being biological parents.) It is American society's preoccupation with genes that leads some to surmise that reproductive technology must inevitably lead to eugenics. It is thus the social context and not just the availability of reproductive technology that gives some credence to the fear that reproductive technology may ultimately produce unsavory consequences.

As we work to create a social policy position on reproductive technology, we shall have to deal with three questions:

Who will have control over reproductive decision making—the state, the medical profession, or the individual?

Will we embrace a genetic or a social vision of parenthood?

Will we focus our efforts on trying to produce the best people free of genetic deficits, or will we embrace a perspective that emphasizes society's responsibility to the welfare of all people?

The most beneficial policies will be, not those specifically directed at the new reproductive technologies, but those that modify the general social context: focusing attention on the welfare of children rather than on reproduction exclusively, fostering a social rather than a biogenetic definition of parenthood, promoting greater opportunities for women, reforming medical institutions to incorporate more humane values, and providing more social support for individuals and families generally. With regard to reproduction specifically, we should promote policies that will offer the maximum number of reproductive choices.

I also advocate specific reforms in the delivery of infertility services: instituting guidelines governing programs' reporting of success rates, creating mechanisms to ensure equal access to infertility treatment, and establishing regulations for the use of particular technologies.[22] I support legislation both requiring IVF clinics to provide prospective clients with accurate information about the success rates of specific clinics and establishing a uniform format for presenting such data.

To insure more equitable access to infertility services, I support the passage of legislation requiring insurance companies to cover the cost of infertility treatment. I am in favor of modifying the Federal Medicaid Program to include reimbursement for infertility services. Infertility services should also be made available to veterans. Family planning agencies are currently required to provide rudimentary infertility assistance, but family planning legislation should be amended to increase the level of help for infertility provided by these agencies. I am also in favor of requiring that infertility clinics devote a certain proportion of their activities to attending to the treatment needs of the poor and near-poor on a pro bono basis.

To slow down the commercialization of reproduction, I advocate banning the sale of human embryos, eggs, and sperm and outlawing commercial surrogacy.[23] I support establishment of a legal principle for settling custody disputes: the right of the gestational woman (that is, she who carries a child) should have precedence over the rights of those who have supplied eggs or sperm.

Wherever possible, public policy should promote the idea that the essence of parenthood is to be found in caring for a child rather than in having genetic links to a child. Adoption legislation should be modified to make adoption more open and therefore a more attractive option for birthmothers. Custody laws should be modified to make it easier to provide adoptive homes for children currently in foster care.

The debate over IVF and other reproductive technologies will continue. It is important that participants in this debate not lose sight of the anguished struggle of infertile couples to become parents. A more nuanced and sensitive understanding of the experience of infertile couples and of the dilemma in which they find themselves, such as that which I have tried to provide in this book, cannot help but improve the quality of this debate.

APPENDIX

INTERVIEW GUIDE
Social and Emotional Aspects of Infertility

1. When did you first begin to try to have children?
2. When did you become aware that you were having difficulties with childbearing?
   a. What made you aware?
   b. What kinds of problems did you have?
   c. Do you think of yourself as infertile?
3. Have you sought medical treatment for this problem?
   a. If yes,
      (1) Describe your treatment history.
      (2) At what point in treatment are you now?
      (3) Do you have a definite diagnosis?
      (4) What treatments are you considering for the future?
   b. If no, why have you not sought treatment?
4. If you have been through medical treatment, please describe your experience with it.
   a. Your relationship with physicians.
   b. Your experience with hospitals.
   c. What was the outcome?
   d. What are your most significant positive and negative memories?
5. Have you considered adoption?
   a. Have you been successful?
   b. What made you choose adoption?
   c. Why have you decided against adoption?

6. Please describe to me your personal emotional reaction to your childbearing difficulties.
   a. What was your immediate reaction?
   b. Did your feelings change over time?
   c. Has it brought you closer together or farther apart as a couple?
   d. How has it affected your sex life?
7. Have you spoken with close friends or family about these difficulties or your treatment experiences?
   a. If not, why not?
   b. Did they understand?
   c. What was their reaction?
   d. Did it change your relationships any?
8. (If children in the home) Do you think your childbearing difficulties have had any effects on your relationship with your children? Is your parenting different than it would have been?
9. Are there special ways that you cope with childbearing difficulties or their treatment?
   a. Are there activities that compensate for childbearing for you?
   b. Have you withdrawn from normal activities at all?
   c. Have you sought professional counseling?
   d. Are you involved with a support group (such as Resolve)?
10. In general, would you say your childbearing difficulties have affected the way you live your life?
    a. Major decisions (moving, changing jobs, etc.)
    b. Orientation (work vs. family vs. leisure)
    c. Views (religious, political, social)
11. Do you ever ask yourself, Why has this happened to me? How do you answer?

NOTES

CHAPTER ONE

1. Schneider and Conrad 1983.

2. Bergman 1938:50; Moose 1911:96; Pasternak 1972:60. I am not aware of any cultures where having no daughters is equated with being childless, but some matrilineal societies, such as the Asian Khasi (Gurdon 1907:85) and the African Bemba (Richards 1956:112), definitely prefer daughters.

3. For Korea, see Griffis 1882:259, 256. For Taiwan, see Pasternak 1972:243; Sung 1975:36; Wolf 1972:22, 172. For African Hausa, see Smith 1959:21. For Iban, see Freeman 1955:7. For Objibwa, see Hilger 1951:33.

4. For Tiv, see Bohannon and Bohannon 1969:74. For Dogon, see Parin, Morgenthaler, and Parin-Matthes 1963:123. For Ganda, see Roscoe 1911:46. For Kurds, see Masters 1953:231. For Tucano, see Silva 1962:418.

5. Rosenblatt et al. 1973:224.

6. See Greer (1984) for a discussion of childless women in society. In some societies, such as the Ashanti of Africa (Christensen 1954:63) and the Kapauku of Papua, New Guinea (Pospisil 1958:175), a woman who has borne no children has the right to divorce her husband. Pospisil argues that in the context of polygyny this makes sense because the husband is free to take another wife but the wife is not free to take another husband.

7. For the Greeks, see Lee 1953:42. For Polish peasants, see Benet 1951:91. For Truk islanders, see Gladwin and Sarason 1953:417. For Klamath Indians, see Pearsall 1950:339B. For the Ashanti, see Christensen 1954:63. For Tikopia, see Firth 1940:485. For Hopi, see Talayevsa 1942:269. For Amayra, see Buechler and Buechler 1971:20.

8. It will be noted that, in many crosscultural examples I present below, cultural explanations of infertility tend to hold the infertile responsible for their own suffering. I address this issue in some detail in Chapter 7. For Ganda, see Mair 1934:38; for Dogon, see Calame-Griaule 1986:680; for Ashanti, see Field 1970:171; for Trukese, see Fischer 1963:529; for Amhara, see Messing 1957:427.

9. For Somali, see Galaal 1968:20; for Toradja, see Adriani and Kruyt 1950:109; for Ashanti, see Field 1970:121; for Ndembu, see Turner 1967, 1968, 1975; for Pawnee, see Dorsey and Murie 1940:92; for Poles, see Benet 1950:91.

10. For Bemba, see Richards 1956:33; for Aowin, see Ebin 1982.

11. For Taiwanese, see Wolf and Huang 1980:212; for Dogon, see Pern 1982:21; for Trukese, see Gladwin and Sarason 1953:2; for Toradja, see Adriani and Kruyt 1951:426.

12. Stein 1989; Payer 1988.

13. This issue is addressed at greater length in Chapter 7.

14. Martin 1987; Riessman 1983; Rothman 1989; Todd 1982.

15. Turner 1967, 1968, 1969, 1975. See especially Turner 1968:302; Turner 1967:361, 12.

16. Degler 1980. Among the first contemporary historians to draw attention to the nineteenth-century ideological view that women are naturally suited to occupy a different "sphere" than men was Nancy Cott (1977).

17. Lasch 1977.

18. Cancian 1987; Komarovsky 1962; Mornell 1979; Rainwater, Coleman, and Handel 1959; Rubin 1976, 1983; Shostak 1969; Swain 1989.

19. Rubin 1983.

20. The interplay between the contemporary institution of the family and the experience of infertility is explored in Chapters 3, 5, and 6.

21. Starr 1982. Conrad and Schneider 1980a; I discuss the concept of medicalization in greater detail in Chapter 2. Preston 1981.

22. See, for example, Ehrenreich and Ehrenreich 1970; Illich 1976; Navarro 1976; Waitzkin 1983.

23. Starr 1982.

24. Mechanic 1968; Todd 1989.

25. Mishler et al. 1981; Zola 1983.

26. The relationship between contemporary medical institutions and the experience of infertility is the major focus of Chapters 2 and 4.

27. Bellah et al. 1985.

28. Berger 1967.

29. I emphasize the relationship between questions of meaning and the experience of infertility in Chapter 7.

30. The other interviewers were Thomas A. Leitko and Karen L. Porter. I have reported upon this other research project in Greil and Leitko (1985), Greil and Porter (1988), and Leitko and Greil (1985).

31. Throughout this discussion of research design, I write in the first person to keep the narrative simpler and clearer. In actuality, Thomas A. Leitko was intimately involved in this project in its early stages and participated fully in making all important decisions concerning research design.

32. Throughout the text, I cite research that is relevant to the particular issue under discussion. Here I mention only systematic reviews of the research literature. Recent reviews of the literature include Cook 1987; Dennerstein and Morse 1988; Martin Matthews and Matthews 1986; Morse and Van Hall 1987; Shapiro 1988.

33. For symbolic interaction, see Blumer 1969; for grounded theory, see Glazer and Strauss 1967.

34. See, for example, Miall 1985, 1986; Olshansky 1987; Sandelowski 1988; Sandelowski and Jones 1986; Sandelowski and Pollock 1986; Woollett 1985.

35. Bernard 1972. For marital misperceptions, see Ballwig 1969; Bernard 1972; Heer 1962; Monroe et al. 1985; Scanzoni 1965; Spitze and Huber 1982; Van Es and Shingi 1972; Wilkening and Morrison 1963.

36. Bernstein, Potts, and Mattox 1985; Freeman et al. 1985; Link and Darling 1986; Mahlstedt, MacDuff, and Bernstein 1987; McEwen, Costello, and Taylor 1987; Sabatelli, Meth, and Gavazzi 1988; Van Keep and Schmidt-Elmendorf 1975.

37. The difference between wives' and husbands' estimates confirm Bernard's (1972) observations about his and hers marriages.

38. Mosher 1982.

39. For clinic-based samples of women, see Miall 1985, 1986; Sandelowski 1988; Sandelowski and Jones 1986; Sandelowski and Pollock 1986; Woollett 1985. For samples including blacks and lower-SES women, see Sandelowski and Jones 1986.

40. Again, this difference may perhaps be evidence of his and hers marriages (Bernard 1972).

41. Miall 1985, 1986.

CHAPTER TWO

1. Mosher 1987:42–43.

2. Menning 1982.

3. Ryder and Westoff 1971:317; Hendershot 1984. Based on a sample drawn from a group Ob/Gyn practice, Page (1989:573) estimates that of English couples 28 percent have experienced infertility at some point in their lives.

4. Hirsch and Mosher 1987.

5. Kalmuss 1987; Hirsch and Mosher 1987; Mosher 1982.

6. For health, see Dougherty 1988; Graham and Reeder 1979; Kitagawa and Hauser 1973; Ries 1985; Syme and Berkman 1976. For access to health care, see Aday, Anderson, and Fleming 1980; Anderson and Anderson 1979; Davis and Rowland 1987; Dougherty 1988; Ries 1987; Riessman 1974; Ross and Duff 1983.

7. Collins et al. 1983; Dor, Hamber, and Rabau 1977; Hull et al. 1985; Insler, Potashnik, and Glassner 1981; Katayama et al. 1979; Kliger 1984; Raymont, Arronet, and Arrata 1969; Templeton and Penney 1982; Thomas and Forest 1980; Verkauf 1983. All data in this section that deal with the incidence of various types of reproductive impairments come from these sources.

It may surprise readers unfamiliar with medical statistics to note how inexact data on the incidence of different medical conditions related to infertility really are. At present, it is impossible to say with any real degree of precision just what proportion of infertile couples have a specific type of reproductive impairment. Estimates of the incidence of different impairments have typically been based on samples of people who have presented themselves for treatment at a single infertility treatment center. Because there has never been a study of the incidence of reproductive impairments within a randomly selected population, we have no way of knowing whether people who seek treatment for infertility are typical of all infertile people. In fact, there is good reason to suspect that they are atypical because those who seek treatment are so different in their social characteristics from those who do not (Hirsch and Mosher 1987).

Furthermore, it is impossible to say whether the same social selection factors operate at all infertility clinics, a point perhaps best explicated with the help of an example. Studies have reported that problems with the Fallopian tubes may be the underlying biomedical cause of infertility in anywhere from 12 to 86 percent of infertile couples (Belsey and Ware 1986:638). What are we to make of these facts: one clinic reports that of its patients 12 percent have tubal problems while another reports that of its patients 86 percent have tubal problems? Is the difference due to national or regional differences in the prevalence of tubal problems? Is it due to national or regional differences in the tendency to be *bothered* by certain types of problems? Does one clinic have a reputation for dealing especially well or especially poorly with tubal problems? Do the investigators at one clinic have special interest or expertise in tubal problems?

Another problem in interpreting statistics stems from the tendency of most studies to report only one principle diagnosis for each infertile couple studied. For many infertile couples more than one factor conditions their infertility. Thus, the tendency to report only the principle diagnosis may result in underreporting certain conditions. Moreover, the decision about which of several problems is the principle one may be influenced as much by the research interests and treatment philosophies of the investigators as by the characteristics of the patients.

A third problem in interpreting statistics on types of reproductive impairments stems from researchers' lack of a common scheme for classifying reproductive impairments, a deficiency that makes it difficult to compare studies.

8. Miall 1985, 1986; Simons 1984.

9. U.S. Congress 1988:117.

10. Collins et al. 1984: 529; Insler, Potashnik, and Glassner 181:171; Kliger 1984:142; Verkauf 1983:178.

11. Davajan and Mishell 1986:384; Kliger 1984:43; Thomas and Forrest 1980; Verkauf 1983:178.

12. Collins et al. 1983.

13. Behrman and Patton 1988:6; Shapiro 1988.

14. One easy way to document this trend is to glance at the number of articles dealing with infertility listed each year in the *Reader's Guide to Periodical Literature*. In the decade prior to 1978, a total of eighteen popular articles on infertility appeared; but in 1978 alone, sixteen infertility articles were published, and on average thirteen articles a year have been published since 1978.

15. Mosher 1987.

16. Rindfuss, Bumpass, and St. John 1980; Rindfuss and St. John 1983; Wilkie 1981.

17. Hirsch and Mosher 1987.

18. U.S. Congress 1988:5.

19. Ibid., 55.

20. Conrad and Schneider 1980a.

21. Ehrenreich and English 1979; Tyack 1974.

22. Conrad and Schneider 1980b.

23. For medical model, see Conrad and Schneider 1980a:35; for analogy to machine, see Osherson and AmaraSingham 1981. For inorganic causes, see Comaroff and Maguire 1986; Conrad and Kerns 1986:7. For diseased organ, see Fisher and Todd 1983; Mizrahi 1986; Scully 1980; Wright 1982.

24. Parsons 1958.

25. Crawford 1986; Herzlich and Pierret 1987; Knowles 1977.

26. Charmaz 1983; Herzlich and Pierret 1987; Zola 1972.

27. For cure, see Fisher and Todd 1983; for acute illness, see Charmaz 1983.

28. Fisher 1988; Fisher and Todd 1983; Mishler 1984; Mizrahi 1986; West 1984).

29. For women's behavior, see Corea 1977; Ehrenreich and English 1979; Fisher 1988; Rothman 1986; 1989; Scully 1980; Todd 1989. For birth, see Arney 1982; Leavitt 1986; Summey and Hurst 1986; Wertz and Wertz 1977. For gynecology, see Scully 1980.

30. Bell 1987; Clarke 1988; Martin 1987; Riessman 1983; Rothman 1989; Todd 1982.

31. Cypress 1984:19.

32. Riessman 1983:14.

33. Summey and Hurst 1986.

34. Clarke 1988.

35. Lewis 1986:136.

36. Harris 1950:179.

37. For Children's Bureau, see Ladd-Taylor 1986:66, 68, 164; for experimental therapy, see Sandelowski 1989: 8; for doctor shopping, see *Science Digest* 1956:50.

38. Lewis 1986:139.

39. Tilt 1881:280.

40. McGregor 1986:124.

41. Baldy 1894:127.

42. Riessman 1983:6.

43. Starr 1982.

44. For herbal remedies, see Fox 1966:77–79; for Dewees's advice, see Radbill 1976:28; for Pinkham's Compound, see Stage 1979:127; for magic pebbles, see Gebhard 1976:97.

45. Haraven 1977:62.

46. Haraven 1984.

47. For older children, see Zelizer 1985; for infants, see Dosch 1910:31.

48. Gruhn and Kazer 1989.

49. Clarke 1988:16.

50. Bell 1987.

51. For nature, see Simons 1988:21; for emotional origin, see Ehrenreich and English 1979:250.

52. Brown 1986:359; Holman and Hammond 1988:359.

53. Gomel et al., 1986:2.

54. Aral and Cates 1983; Scritchfield 1989.

55. Aral and Cates 1983; Scritchfield 1989.

56. Ubell 1990:15.

57. Medical Research International and the Society of Assisted Reproductive Technology 1989.

58. Katz and Katz 1987:401.

59. For unwed mothers, see Feinberg 1984:43; for decreased adoptions, see Plumez 1980:34; for leveling of decrease, see Bachrach 1986:245–246.

60. The total fertility rate is the number of births that 1,000 women would have in their lifetime if, at each year of age, they experienced the birth rates occurring in that specific year. For high, see U.S. Bureau of the Census 1975:50; for low, see U.S. Bureau of the Census 1989:64.

61. For 1957, see U.S. Bureau of the Census 1975:49; for 1975, see U.S. Bureau of the Census 1989:61.

62. For more gynecologists, see U.S. Congress 1988:5. For decline in visits, see Gonzalez and Emmons 1988:68; Reynolds and Ohsfeldt 1984:64. For reasons to specialize, see Scritchfield 1989:105.

63. For publicity, see Pfeffer 1987; for repeatable therapies, see Talbert 1985:11.

64. Rothman 1982:121–122.

65. Hubbard 1981; Lorber 1988; Menning 1977.

66. For chronic, see Flemming 1984; Greil, Leitko, and Porter 1988; Greil 1989. For intrusion, see Strauss et al. 1984:11–17.

67. Infertile couples are likely to schedule sex for several reasons. First, couples try to ensure they will have intercourse when the wife is likely to be ovulating. Because the couple put the dots on the BBT chart, they are usually constantly aware of where they stand in the wife's cycle—whether a particular day is a "good" time for

sex. Second, the number of sperm in a man's ejaculate will be greater if intercourse is not too frequent. Physicians generally suggest that a couple wait thirty-six to forty-eight hours after intercourse before engaging in intercourse again. Third, frequent ejaculation leads to a more rapid replenishing of a man's sperm. Thus, some couples make it a point to engage in intercourse at regular intervals even when the woman is not in the fertile stage of her cycle.

68. Daly 1988; Greil 1989; Greil, Leitko, and Porter 1989.

CHAPTER THREE

1. For timetables, see Roth 1963. For age norms, see Hogan and Astone 1986; Modell 1980, 1989; Neugarten, Moore, and Lowe 1965; Plath and Ikeda 1976. For predictability, see Hareven 1977; Kohli 1986; Modell 1989.

2. Hogan and Astone 1986.

3. For normative, see Busfield and Paddon 1977; Gormly, Gormly, and Weiss 1987; Knaub, Eversoll, and Voss 1983; Russo 1976. For deviant, see Blake 1979; Callan 1983; Houseknecht 1979, 1987; Jamison, Franzini, and Kaplan 1979; Miall 1985, 1986; Ory 1978; Veevers 1979, 1980.

4. Blake 1979; Gormly, Gormly, and Weiss 1987; Buchman 1989. Gormly, Gormly, and Weiss found that 55.6 percent of their female subjects but only 32.1 percent of their male subjects said, in response to an open-ended question, that they saw having children as a way of achieving adult status. Christine Fry's (1983) sample of 242 adults saw twenty-six as the age at which people "ought" to have preschool age children in the home.

5. Burgoyne 1987:49.

6. Miall 1987; Schneider 1968.

7. Risman (1987) refers to this position as "microstructuralism."

8. Fisher and Todd 1983; Herzlich and Pierret 1987; Martin 1987; Osherson and AmaraSingham 1981; Rothman 1989.

9. Woollett (1985) also mentions the theme of "body failure."

10. The term "spoiled identity" is borrowed from Goffman (1963). He uses the term to describe a situation in which the sense of self that one attempts to maintain and display to others has been discredited by the fact that the individual in question possesses certain stigmatizing characteristics. I deal with the question of infertility as social stigma in Chapter 6.

11. Other authors who emphasize the theme of "feeling defective" include Cook (1987), Mahlstedt (1985), and Mazor (1984). Victor Callan (1987) did not find that the female IVF patients he studied scored significantly different on measures of psychological well-being from the voluntarily childless women and the mothers to

which he compared them, but he did find that they were significantly less satisfied with themselves and their accomplishments.

12. Lerner 1980.

13. Kathy Charmaz (1983), in a discussion of the effects of chronic illness on sense of self, also highlights the fact that sufferers often share cultural values that hold them responsible for their own condition.

14. For marriage, see Bernard 1972. For infertility, see Freeman et al. (1985), who found, in a study of 200 IVF couples, that 48 percent of the wives but only 15 of the husbands rated infertility as the worst experience in their lives. Sabatelli, Meth, and Gavazzi developed an "Infertility Adjustment Scale" and administered it to fifty-two infertile wives and twenty-nine husbands. The husbands scored significantly higher than the wives. Other studies have suggested that infertile women express more feelings of anger and helplessness (Mahlstedt, MacDuff, and Bernstein 1987), more feelings of disappointment (Van Keep and Schmidt-Elmendorf 1975), a greater sense of a decrease in self-confidence (Sabatelli, Meth, and Gavazzi 1988), less self-esteem (Bernstein, Potts, and Mattox 1985), and lower life satisfaction (Link and Darling 1986) than infertile men. None of these studies reported on which partners in their samples had reproductive impairments.

Lalos et al. (1985) studied twenty-four infertile couples in which the wives had had surgery for tubal damage and found, not surprisingly, that the wives reported being more affected by infertility than their husbands. McEwan, Costello, and Taylor (1987) and Raval et al. (1987) both found in studies of clinic samples of infertile couples that women evidenced higher levels of psychological stress than men, no matter which partner had the reproductive impairment. In a study of 843 infertile couples, Connolly, Edelmann, and Cooke (1987) found that wives scored marginally higher on a "distress" scale than did their husbands, regardless of which partner had the reproductive impairment. They also found, however, that both husbands and wives reported more marital problems in cases involving a male reproductive impairment. Miall (1985, 1986) found that involuntarily childless women felt that more stigma is attached to male infertility than to female infertility, but she interviewed only women.

Van Keep and Schmidt-Elmendorff (1975) asked members of seventy-five infertile couples whether they thought infertility was worse for wives or for husbands. Husbands were much more likely to say infertility was worse for the wife (72 percent); 45 percent of the wives gave this answer. Only one husband and one wife said infertility was a bigger disappointment for the husband.

15. Only a few research studies have addressed the question of how responses to infertility may be affected by which partner has the reproductive impairment. Daniluk, Leader, and Taylor (1987) found in a study of forty-three infertile couples that the partner with the reproductive impairment was more likely to experience

higher levels of stress. Charlene Miall (1986) has observed that involuntarily child-less wives without reproductive impairments are less likely than those with reproductive impairments to feel rapport with other infertile women. Snarey et al. (1987) found better marital outcomes for infertile couples when both husband and wife had reproductive impairments than for couples where only one spouse had a reproductive impairment, but this relationship was not statistically significant. The same authors did not find medical diagnosis to have any significant effects on the psychological development of the infertile men they studied. Bernstein, Mattox, and Kellner (1988) found no relationship between diagnosis and scores on a test of psychological functioning. Connolly, Edelmann, and Cook (1987) noted that male infertility led to higher rates of reported marital problems for both husbands and wives.

16. Miall 1985:395–396. The term "master status" was introduced to sociology by Hughes (1945).

17. DeJong et al. 1984; Hanson et al. 1984.

18. Cozby 1973; Davidson and Duberman 1982; Fitzpatrick and Indvik 1982; Morgan 1976; Parelman 1983; Peplau and Gordon 1985; Rubin 1983.

19. The term, "feeling rules" comes from Hochschild (1983). For a good discussion of emotional norms as they relate to gender, see Shields (1987).

20. For emotional women, see Cancian and Gordon 1988; Shields and Koster 1989. For expectations, see Allen and Haccoun 1976; Allen and Hamsher 1974; Balswick and Avertt 1977; Brody 1985; Caldwell and Peplau 1982; Shimanoff 1983. For two spheres, see Degler 1980. For divided marriages, see Rubin 1976, 1983. Helpful discussions of the emotional division of labor within the family may also be found in Daniels (1987), Hocschild (1989), and Riessman (1990).

21. Cancian 1987; Rubin 1976, 1983.

22. For parent role, see Busfield 1987; Hogan and Astone 1986. For mandate, see Russo 1976.

23. I am grateful to Judith N. Lasker for reminding me of this point.

24. U.S. Congress 1988:55.

25. Martin 1987; Riessman 1983.

26. Stack 1974.

27. Halle 1984.

28. Goody 1976.

29. Hoffman and Manis 1979. Note that although reasons having to do with family and self-continuity are not especially popular among either men or women, they are certainly more popular among men.

30. Collins 1979.

31. Zelizer 1985.

32. Cancian 1987.

33. When I suggest this, I do not mean to imply that men have not also been nurturing caretakers for children. See, for example, Degler (1980) and Demos (1986).

34. Crowe 1985; Lasker and Borg 1987; Lorber 1988; Stanworth 1987.

35. Lasker and Borg 1987:16; Stanworth 1987:22.

36. Crowe 1985; Lasker and Borg 1987; Lorber and Greenfield 1989.

37. For willing wives, see Greil, Leitko, and Porter 1988; Lasker 1988. For wifely agreement, see Lorber 1989. For patriarchal bargains, see Kandiyoti 1988.

38. Arditti 1985; Crowe 1985; Lasker 1988; Rothman 1984; Rowland 1987.

CHAPTER FOUR

1. Cook 1987; Lorber and Greenfield 1989; Matthews and Martin Matthews 1986; Mazor 1979; McCormick 1980; Platt, Ficher, and Silver 1973; Woollett 1985. Paulson et al. (1988) found no appreciable differences between the infertile women and fertile controls on measures of personality, depression, anxiety, or self-concept; but they did discover that infertile women were more likely to see themselves as affected by forces outside their control. Almost half of the ninety-four participants in an IVF program who filled out a questionnaire distributed by Mahlstedt, MacDuff, and Bernstein (1987) said that most stressful aspect of infertility was feeling a loss of control.

2. Aral and Cates 1983; Scritchfield 1989.

3. Woollett 1985:476.

4. Cf. Miall 1986.

5. In this section we have been listening to wives describe physicians who were unwilling to begin infertility treatment. It is not clear how we are to reconcile these accounts with the evidence (presented in Chapter 2) that more and more gynecologists are moving into the area of infertility. It may be the case that, while many gynecologists are becoming interested in infertility, many still are not. It is also possible that wives' accounts describe the past behavior of physicians and that their behavior now has changed. Wives were interviewed in 1985 and 1986. At the time they were interviewed, they had been dealing with infertility for an average of 6.7 years. Because the encounters they are describing took place early in their infertility careers, their accounts may reveal more about these gynecologists' approaches to infertility ten years ago than about their current approaches.

6. Riessman 1983.

7. It should be noted here that the behavior of Jean's physician cannot be interpreted as simply an attempt to have Jean wait the medically approved period before beginning her workup. Jean's doctor waited to begin her workup until Jean had been

trying to conceive for almost two years, nearly twice as long as the generally accepted medical trial period.

8. Lorber 1988:17.

9. Freidson 1970; Mishler et al. 1981; Parsons 1958; Todd 1989; Waitzkin and Waterman 1974; Zola 1972.

10. For power imbalance, see Freidson 1970. For physicians' control, see Fisher 1988; Fisher and Todd 1983; Korsch and Negrete 1972; Mishler 1984; Todd 1989; West 1984. For typical interview, see Korsch and Negrete 1972. For doctors' questions, see West 1984. For female patients, see Corea 1977; Ehrenreich and English 1979; Fisher 1988; Rothman 1986, 1989; Scully 1980; Todd 1989. For patients' dissatisfaction, see Francis, Korsch, and Morris 1969; Korsch and Negrete 1972; Mechanic 1968; Todd 1989. For changing physicians, see Mechanic 1968.

11. Lorber and Greenfield 1989; Pirie 1988.

12. For patients as active, see Arluke 1980; Conrad 1985, 1987; Hayes-Bautista 1976; McGuire 1988; Pirie 1988; Roth 1972; Singer, Davison, and Gerdes 1988. For factors, see Zola 1983.

13. Hayes-Bautista 1976.

14. Roth 1972.

15. McGuire 1988:194, 198.

16. Owens and Read (1984:15) report that some infertile women who responded to their questionnaire asserted that they too had taken an active role in influencing the course of their infertility investigations. Owens and Read speculate that those who take greater initiative may ultimately be more satisfied with their treatment experiences.

17. Woollett 1985:477.

18. Danziger 1986.

19. Again, we find support for Riessman's (1983) assertion that women are often active supporters of the process of medicalization. In a British study of 387 infertile women, Owens and Read (1984:16) found that many of their respondents, too, were dissatisfied with the speed at which infertility investigations progressed.

20. Although it is impossible merely on the basis of patients' recollections about the progress of their infertility treatment to make a definitive judgment about the quality of care they received, it does seem to be the case that some gynecologists did depart from generally accepted procedures. Janet had been in treatment for eight years, but none of her doctors had ever performed a laparoscopy. Cathy's gynecologist prescribed clomiphene citrate in the absence of any clear indication of an ovulatory problem. Debby took clomiphene citrate for three years without any apparent effect. It is, of course, possible that patients' accounts may be incomplete or incorrect in some details, so I hesitate to attribute too much significance to this kind of data.

21. Owens and Read (1984:11) found that the vast majority of their infertile respondents in England felt that the medical professionals who had treated them had not paid sufficient attention to the emotional and psychological aspects of their problem.

22. Charmaz 1983, 1987; Strauss et al. 1984.

23. Stamell 1983:32.

24. Studies by Lalos et al. (1985) and Olshansky (1987) also found that few, if any, infertile couples find the child-free option acceptable.

25. For the infertile's difficulty conceding permanent condition, see Crowe 1985; Greil 1989; Lasker and Borg 1987; Rothman 1984; Rowland 1987; Scritchfield 1989. For another step, see Crowe 1985; Greil 1989; Lasker and Borg 1987; Scritchfield 1989.

26. In Chapter 2, I noted that, in general, contemporary gynecologists have an "interventionist orientation."

27. Lasker and Borg 1987:64.

28. Bury 1982.

29. My term "status blockage" is similar to the term "role blocking" employed by Matthews and Martin Matthews (1986).

30. Matthews and Martin Matthews 1986; Turner 1966; Daly 1988. See also Margarete Sandelowski (1987, 1988) who, I think, speaks to this same issue when she says that "ambiguity" is a central feature of the experience of infertile women.

CHAPTER FIVE

1. Cancian and Gordon 1988.

2. For expectations, see Shields 1987. For wifely oversight of emotion, see Cancian and Gordon 1988; Daniels 1987; Riessman 1990. For negative emotions, see Shimanoff 1985. For wifely orchestration, see Markman 1984. For wifely sensitivity, see Blumstein and Schwartz 1983; Huston and Ashmore 1986; Krokoff 1987; Thompson and Walker 1989. For emotional appeals, see Rubin 1983; Thompson and Walker 1989.

3. For communicative marriage, see Cancian 1987. For American dichotomy, see Caldwell and Peplau 1982; Cancian 1987; Davidson and Duberman 1982; Komarovsky 1974; Rubin 1976, 1983; Swain 1989; Weiss and Lowenthal 1975. For expressiveness, see Allen and Haccoun 1976; Allen and Hamsher 1974; Balswick and Avertt 1977; Brody 1985; Caldwell and Peplau 1982; Cancian 1987; Rubin 1976, 1983; Shimanoff 1985. For self-disclosure, see Cozby 1973; Davidson and Duberman 1982; Fitzpatrick and Indvik 1982; Morgan 1976; Parelman 1983; Peplau and Gordon 1985; Rubin 1976, 1983.

4. For socialization, see Wills, Weiss, and Patterson 1974. For tension, see Cancian 1987; Komarovsky 1962; Mornell 1979; Rainwater, Coleman, and Handel 1959; Rubin 1976, 1983; Shostak 1969; Wills, Weiss, and Patterson 1974.

5. Rubin 1983; Bernard 1972.

6. Greil and Porter 1989.

7. The finding reported by Sabatelli, Meth, and Gavazzi (1988) that husbands' adjustment to infertility was correlated with their wives' anxiety levels also seems to support this interpretation, as does the finding related by Lalos et al. (1985) that the husbands in twenty-four infertile couples were more likely than their wives to report deterioration in the marital relationship.

8. Miall 1985, 1986.

9. In three cases, husbands thought that infertility had strengthened their marital relationships, while their wives either felt that the relationship had become less close (2) or that the relationship was unchanged (1). In four cases, wives felt that the relationship was made closer by infertility, while their husbands either disagreed (1) or were unsure (3). In one case, the wife thought infertility made the marriage less close while her husband did not feel that the marriage had really been affected that much.

10. Berk and Shapiro 1984; Kaufman 1969; Kraft et al. 1980; Mahlstedt 1985; Mazor 1984; Menning 1977, 1979. Berk and Shapiro and Kraft et al. also note that infertility may strengthen some relationships.

11. For marital communication, see Van Keep and Schmidt-Elmendorf 1975:41; for marital satisfaction, see Callan 1987:852. In another study, Sabatelli, Meth, and Gavazzi (1988:340) found a difference of opinion among the fifty-two infertile women and twenty-nine infertile men they studied. On the one hand, 26 percent of the women and 10 percent of the men said that infertility had led to increased satisfaction with their marriages. On the other hand, 22 percent of the women and 18 percent of the men thought infertility had led to a decline in marital satisfaction.

12. Barbarin, Hughes, and Chesler 1985.

13. Van Keep and Schmidt-Elmendorf 1975.

14. For correlation, see Bell and Bell 1972; Blumstein and Schwartz 1983; Carlson 1976; Frank, Anderson, and Rubenstein 1979; Gebhard 1966; Greenblat 1983; Hunt 1970; Klagsbrun 1985; Patton and Waring 1985; Perlman and Abramson 1982; Schenk, Pfrang, and Rausche 1983; Udry 1974; Wallin and Clark 1964. Patton and Waring, however, are careful to point out that the correlation between sexual satisfaction and intimacy is by no means perfect. See especially Blumstein and Schwartz 1983:201.

15. Cited in Klagsbrun 1985:117.

16. Blumstein and Schwartz 1983.

17. Berk and Shapiro 1984; Burgwyn 1981; Freeman et al. 1985; Golden 1983; Kaufman 1969; Lalos et al. 1985; Greil, Leitko, and Porter 1989; Mazor 1979, 1980,

1984; Menning 1977, 1979; Raval et al. 1987; Reed 1987; Sabatelli, Meth, and Gavazzi 1988; Walker 1978. Only a few published research studies attempt to assess the effects of infertility on sexual relationships. In a study of fifty-two infertile women and twenty-nine infertile men, Sabatelli, Meth, and Gavazzi (1988:340) found that 55 percent of the men and 56 percent of the women they studied said that infertility had resulted in a lower frequency of sexual intercourse, while 42 percent of the men and 59 percent of the women said that their sexual satisfaction had decreased as a result of infertility. In a study of forty-seven infertile couples, Raval et al. (1987:231) found that, while women report more relationship problems resulting from infertility than do men, the problems that men do report seem to center around issues of sexuality. See especially Berk and Shapiro 1984:43.

18. Kaufman (1969) also stresses the impact of scheduled sex for sexual satisfaction among infertile couples.

19. For sex as procreation, see Mazor (1984); for mechanical sex, see Menning (1977).

20. Loss of privacy is also mentioned by Fenton and Lifchez (1980) and Matthews and Martin Matthews (1986). Other authors who note the disruptive role of the BBT regimen for marital and sexual relationships include Bullock (1974), Debrovner and Shubin-Stein (1976), and Kaufman (1969).

21. Kaufman 1985.

22. Blumstein and Schwartz 1983.

CHAPTER SIX

1. Albrecht 1976; Chaiklin and Warfield 1977; Charmaz 1983, 1987; Davis 1961; Gussow and Tracy 1968; Scott 1978.

2. Albrecht, Walker, and Levy 1982; Friedson 1966; Goffman 1963; Gussow and Tracy 1968; Hanks and Poplin 1981; Schneider and Conrad 1983; Scambler 1984.

3. Miall 1985, 1986. See especially Miall 1985:391.

4. For Duncan, see McLane and McLane 1969:866; for poor hygiene, see Macomber 1924:67; for higher education, see Sturgis 1957.

5. Sandelowski 1989:442–443.

6. Ford 1945:101. For blacks, see Billingsley 1968:59; Rohrer and Edmonson 1960:113. For Mormons, see Fife and Fife 1966:103; Sorenson 1976:20. For U.S. couples, see Miall 1985, 1986; Sandelowski 1989. For Poles, see Benet 1951:91; for Serbs, see Erlich 1966:303; for Jews, see Zborowski and Herzog 1952:310. For Africa, see Collier and Rosaldo 1981:304; for Ashanti, see Rattray 1923:67. For Cagaba, see Tschopik 1951:20.

7. Sandelowski and Jones (1986) call infertility an "invisible stigma"; and Simons (1984) calls it an "invisible handicap." For condition, see Goffman 1963. For

epileptics, see Schneider and Conrad 1983. Keeping this stigma secret is, of course, not true for those who have adopted a child of another race. Such people have, in effect, "gone public" with their infertility.

8. Scambler 1984:215. For epileptics, see Scambler and Hopkins 1985, especially 217.

9. Miall 1985, 1986.

10. Anspach 1979; Levitin 1979; Lorber 1967; Poole, Regoli, and Pogrebin 1986; Rottenberg 1975; Turner 1971.

11. Thoits 1985.

12. For traditional societies, see Poston et al. 1983; Poston and Trent 1984. For Tiv, see Bohannan and Bohannan 1969:74; for Ganda, see Roscoe 1911:46; for Taiwanese, see Wolf and Huang 1980:165; for Thai, see Piker 1975:91; for Dogon, see Parin, Morgenthaler, and Parin-Matthes 1963:170; for Tlingit, see Jones 1944:45; for Iroquois, see Randle 1951:177; for Tzeltal, see Villa Rojas 1969:223-B; for Greeks, see Stephanides 1941:14; for Taiwanese mother-in-law, see Wolf 1972:149.

13. Erlich 1966.

14. Grabill, Kiser, and Whelpton 1973:392.

15. Mattesich 1979:300.

16. Lynd and Lynd 1929:131, 1982:164.

17. Gramling and Forsythe 1987. The ideas expressed in this paragraph owe much to discussions I have had with Judith N. Lasker.

18. Friedson 1966; Lorber 1967.

19. Several other writers have called attention to strained relationships between the infertile and the fertile world. The most thorough treatment of this theme is to be found in Sandelowski and Jones (1986). In a study of fifty-two infertile wives and twenty-nine of their husbands, Sabatelli, Meth, and Gavazzi (1988) found that 49 percent of the wives and 24 percent of the husbands said that contact with their friends decreased as a result of infertility. Furthermore, 43 percent of the wives and 17 percent of the husbands reported that their comfort with friends had decreased. Lalos et al. (1985) reported that their sample of twenty-four tubal surgery patients and their husbands did not feel that their friends and relatives had been supportive.

20. Sandelowski and Jones (1986:177) call this strategy "putting on a happy face."

21. Thoits 1985; Borkman 1984.

22. Gartner and Riessman 1984.

23. Leerhsen 1990:50.

CHAPTER SEVEN

1. Bury 1982.

2. Kushner 1981.

3. Bulman and Wortman 1977:358.

4. For religion, see Berger 1967; Geertz 1968; Greeley 1972; Kelley 1977; Luckmann 1967. For solutions, see Berger 1967; Geertz 1968; McGuire 1981; Weber 1963.

5. Williams (1984) uses the term "narrative reconstruction" to describe this process of reinterpreting the meaning of one's life in light of a personal tragedy.

6. Shulamit Reinharz (1988) makes a similar point with regard to the experience of miscarriage.

7. In a number of societies, infertility is seen as a result of the violation of sacred norms. For example, the Dogon believe that infertility can be caused by improper treatment of ritual masks (Dieterlen 1941: 244). The Toradja conceptualize infertility as a punishment for not properly serving one's ancestors (Adriani and Kruyt 1951:347). For other peoples, such as the Middle Eastern Amhara (Messing 1957:427) and the Lau of Fiji (Thompson 1940:83), infertility is punishment for promiscuous behavior. The Ashanti (Field 1970:171), the Tiv (Bohannan and Bohannan 1969:69), and the Dogon (Calame-Griaule 1986:680) are three African societies in which infertility is held to be a consequence of quarrelsome marital relations. See especially Ebin 1982:147–149.

8. Weber 1963.

9. Conrad and Schneider 1980a:35.

10. Engel 1977:130.

11. Bulman and Wortman 1977; Comoroff and Maguire 1986; Cook and Wimberly 1983; Greil et al. 1989; Hilbert 1984; Kleinman 1988; Kotarba 1983; Williams 1984.

12. Comoroff and Maguire 1986; see also Herzlich and Pierret 1987. For mine disaster, see Kroll-Smith and Couch 1987. There is a crucial difference between Kroll-Smith and Couch's findings and my own: they found that people did not ask, Why me?, while many people in my sample posed the question but were unable to answer it. Perhaps the collective nature of the situation that Kroll-Smith and Couch describe made the Why me? question unintelligible for the people they studied.

13. The ideas in this and the next several paragraphs were developed as a result of conversations with Per Anderson.

14. Crawford 1986; Glassner 1988; Herzlich and Pierret 1987; Knowles 1977.

15. This idea was suggested to me by Catherine Kohler Riessman.

16. All fifteen wives who spontaneously used transcendent language reported experiencing infertility as meaning threatening. None of the three wives who did not spontaneously use transcendent language experienced infertility as meaning threatening. Of twelve husbands who used transcendent language spontaneously, six (50 percent) experienced infertility as meaning threatening; of ten husbands who did not use transcendent language spontaneously, only two (20 percent) experienced infertility in this light.

Of eleven wives who reported attending religious services on a regular basis, nine (81.9 percent) saw infertility as a threat to meaning; of eleven wives who did not report attending services, six (66.7 percent) saw infertility as meaning threatening. Of nine husbands who attended services regularly, four (44.4 percent) experienced infertility as meaning threatening. Of thirteen nonattenders, three (33.3 percent) husbands saw infertility as a threat to meaning.

17. In the nine cases where the wife had a diagnosed reproductive impairment and the husband did not, four wives (66.7 percent) found infertility threatening at the level of meaning. In the four cases where the husband had a diagnosed reproductive impairment while the wife did not, three wives (75 percent) found infertility threatening at the level of meaning. Among husbands, three of those (75 percent) in the "male reproductive impairment only" situation reported finding infertility threatening at the level of meaning, while three (33.3 percent) of those in the "female reproductive impairment only" group saw infertility as meaning threatening.

18. Of twelve wives who were active in Resolve, eleven (91.7 percent) saw infertility as a threat to meaning. Of the ten wives not active in Resolve, four (40 percent) saw infertility as meaning threatening. Of ten husbands active in Resolve, five (50 percent) saw infertility as meaning threatening; four of the twelve husbands (33.3 percent) not active in Resolve experienced infertility as a threat to meaning.

19. For auto accident victims, see Lehman, Wortman, and Williams 1987; for children with leukemia, see Comaroff and Maguire 1986.

20. Bulman and Wortman 1977:360.

21. For dealing with death, see Cook and Wimberly 1983. For dealing with illness, see Comaroff and Maguire 1986; Hilbert 1984; Kotarba 1983. For the chronic sufferers, see Hilbert 1984; Kotarba 1983.

22. For loss of spouse, see Lehman, Wortman, and Williams 1987. Unfortunately, the authors do not distinguish between parents who lost an only child and those who had surviving children. A study of parents whose children had died as a result of cancer or blood disorders found that the presence of other children in the home effectively strengthened the religious beliefs of parents whose child had died of cancer (Cook and Wimberly 1983:235).

23. Comaroff and Maguire 1986.

CHAPTER EIGHT

1. Hubbard 1981; Lorber 1988; Menning 1977.

2. Some in vitro fertilization clinics do feature couple-centered treatment and an integrated counseling program (cf. Freeman et al. 1985; Haseltine et al. 1985; Kemeter, Eder, and Springer-Kremser 1985). But many couples don't undergo in

vitro fertilization, and those who eventually make their way to IVF clinics have usually spent several years being treated in settings that are not couple-centered and that do not feature routine counseling. Finally, even IVF clinics that do feature counseling tend to assume, without exploring each example, that pursuing a biological child is the best solution to the problem of infertility (Hubbard 1981; Lorber 1988).

3. For general reviews of the political, ethical, and religious literature on reproductive technology, see Donchin (1986), Greil (1989), and Walters (1979). This is, perhaps, the place to point out that not all the so-called new reproductive technologies are all that new. For example, surrogate motherhood, perhaps the most controversial of the "new technologies" currently in use is clearly not the product of any radical advances in medical technology. The only technology involved is AID, which has been in use for about a hundred years. Even IVF is not as new as it seems. Human eggs were successfully fertilized in the United States in the late 1940s, but work was phased out in the 1950s because of a hostile social climate (Lorber 1988).

4. Donchin 1986:124.

5. A good example of this perspective is Andrews (1984).

6. *FerreFax* 1990.

7. As of 1988, six states had passed such legislation: Arkansas, Delaware, Hawaii, Maryland, Massachusetts, and Texas (U.S. Congress 1988:149–151).

8. For examples of conservative approaches to the question of reproductive technology, see the Vatican's "Instruction on Respect for Human Life in Its Origin and on the Dignity of Procreation—Replies to Certain Questions of the Day" (*Origins* 1987) as well as Kass (1971).

9. Falwell 1987.

10. The feminist literature on reproductive technology is quite extensive. A few of the best-known feminist works on this subject are Arditti, Klein, and Minden (1984), Corea (1985), Corea et al. (1987), Overall (1987), Rothman (1986, 1989), Spallone and Steinberg (1987), and Stanworth (1987). Reviews and critiques of the feminist literature on reproductive technology include Franklin and McNeil (1988), Lauritzen (1990), Sandelowski (1989), and Wikler (1986). Of course, "feminism" is not a monolithic perspective, and not all those who consider themselves "feminists" oppose the development of reproductive technology. Laurie B. Andrews, perhaps the best-known representative of the "rights" perspective, considers herself a feminist.

11. Crowe 1985; Rowland 1987.

12. Rothman 1984, 1986, 1989; Sandelowski 1989; Williams 1988.

13. Lauritzen 1990:42.

14. Rothman 1984, 1986, 1989.

15. Dworkin 1983.

16. The high cost of IVF is one example of the exploitation of infertile couples. It

has been argued that hospitals, knowing they can count on infertile couples to make great financial sacrifices to achieve parenthood, charge high fees for IVF as a means of raising revenues to support other services.

17. Riessman 1983.

18. Hubbard 1981; Overall 1987.

19. C.f. Sandelowski 1990.

20. Solomon 1988.

21. See Rothman (1989) for an attempt to formulate a feminist stance on reproductive technology that is sensitive to the concerns of the infertile.

22. For an excellent discussion of policy options regarding infertility, see U.S. Congress (1988).

23. Sherman and Annas 1986.

REFERENCES

Aday, L. A., R. Anderson, and G. V. Fleming. 1980. *Health Care in the U.S.: Equitable for Whom?* Beverly Hills, Calif.: Sage.

Adriani, N., and A. C. Kruyt. 1950. *DeBareé Sprekende Toradjas Van Midden-Celebes (de Oost-Toradjas).* Vol. 1. 2d ed. Amsterdam: Uitgevers Maatschappij.

———. 1951. *DeBareé Sprekende Toradjas Van Midden-Celebes (de Oost-Toradjas).* Vol. 2. 2d ed. Amsterdam: Uitgevers Maatschappij.

Albrecht, G. L. 1976. "Socialization and the Disability Process." In *Disability and Rehabilitation*, ed. G. Albrecht, 3–38 Pittsburgh: University of Pittsburgh Press.

Albrecht, G. L., V. G. Walker, and J. A. Levy. 1982. "Social Distance from the Stigmatized: A Test of Two Theories." *Social Science and Medicine* 16:1319–1327.

Allen, J. G., and D. M. Haccoun. 1976. "Sex Differences in Emotionality: A Multidimensional Approach." *Human Relations* 29:11–720.

Allen, J. G., and J. Hamsher. 1974. "The Development and Validation of Tests of Emotional Styles." *Journal of Consulting and Clinical Psychology* 42:663–668.

Anderson, R., and O. Anderson. 1979. "Trends in the Use of Health Services." In *Handbook of Medical Sociology*, ed. H. E. Freeman, S. Levine, and L. G. Reeder, 371–391. 3d ed. Englewood Cliffs, N.J.: Prentice-Hall.

Andrews, L. B. 1984. *New Conceptions: A Consumer's Guide to the Newest Infertility Treatments, Including In Vitro Fertilization, Artificial Insemination, and Surrogate Motherhood.* New York: St. Martins.

Anspach, R. R. 1979. "From Stigma to Identity Politics: Political Activism Among the Physically Disabled and Former Mental Patients." *Social Science and Medicine* 13:765–773.

Aral, S. O., and W. Cates. 1983. "The Increasing Concern with Infertility: Why Now?" *Journal of the American Medical Association* 250:2327–2331.

Arditti, R. 1985. "Reproductive Engineering and the Social Control of Women." *Radical America* 19:9–26.

Arditti, R., R. D. Klein, and S. Minden, eds. 1984. *Test-Tube Women: What Future for Motherhood?* London: Pandora.

Arluke, A. 1980. "Judging Drugs: Patients' Conceptions of Therapeutic Efficacy in the Treatment of Arthritis." *Human Organization* 39:84–87.

References

Arney, W. 1982. *Power and the Profession of Obstetrics.* Chicago: University of Chicago Press.

Bachrach, C. A. 1986. "Adoption Plans, Adopted Children, and Adoptive Mothers." *Journal of Marriage and the Family* 48:243–253.

Baldy, J. M. 1984. *An American Text-Book of Gynecology, Medical and Surgical, for Practitioners and Students.* Philadelphia: W. B. Saunders.

Ballwig, J. A. 1969. "Husband-Wife Response Similarities on Evaluative and Non-evaluative Survey Questions." *Public Opinion Quarterly* 33:249–254.

Balswick, J., and C. Avertt. 1977. "Differences in Expressiveness: Gender, Interpersonal Orientation, and Perceived Parental Expressiveness as Contributing Factors." *Journal of Marriage and the Family* 39:121–128.

Barbarin, O. A., D. Hughes, and M. A. Chesler. 1985. "Stress, Coping, and Marital Functioning among Parents of Children with Cancer." *Journal of Marriage and the Family* 47:473–480.

Behrman, S. J., and G. W. Patton, Jr. 1988. "Evaluation of Infertility in the 1980s." In *Progress in Infertility*, ed. S. J. Behrman, R. W. Kistner, and G. W. Patton, Jr. 1–22 3d ed. Boston: Little, Brown.

Bell, R. R., and P. L. Bell. 1972. "Sexual Satisfaction Among Married Women." *Medical Aspects of Human Sexuality* 6:136–144.

Bell, S. E. 1987. "Changing Ideas: The Medicalization of Menopause." *Social Science and Medicine* 24:535–542.

Bellah, R. N., R. Madsen, W. M. Sullivan, A. Swindler, and S. M. Tipton. 1985. *Habits of the Heart: Individualism and Commitment in American Life.* Berkeley: University of California Press.

Belsey, M. A., and H. Ware. 1986. "Epidemiological, Social, and Psychosocial Aspects of Infertility." In *Infertility: Male and Female*, ed. V. Insler and B. Lunenfeld, 631–647. Edinburgh: Churchill Livingstone.

Benet, S. 1951. *Song, Dance, and Customs of Peasant Poland.* New York: Roy.

Berger, P. L. 1967. *The Sacred Canopy: Elements of a Sociological Theory of Religion.* Garden City, N.Y.: Doubleday.

Bergman, S. 1938. *In Korean Wilds and Villages.* London: Jack Gifford.

Berk, A. and J. L. Shapiro. 1984. "Some Implications of Infertility on Marital Therapy." *Family Therapy* 11:37–47.

Bernard, J. 1972. *The Future of Marriage.* New York: World.

Bernstein, J., J. H. Mattox, and R. Kellner. 1988. "Psychological Status of Previously Infertile Couples After a Successful Pregnancy." *Journal of Obstetrical Gynecological and Neonatal Nursing* 14:404–408.

Bernstein, J., N. Potts, and J. Mattox. 1985. "Assessment of Psychologic Dysfunction Associated with Infertility." *Journal of Obstetrical and Gynecological and Neonatal Nursing* 14(supp.):63S–66S.

References

Billingsley, A. 1968. *Black Families in White America*. Englewood Cliffs, N.J.: Prentice-Hall.

Blake, J. 1979. "Is Zero Preferred?: American Attitudes Toward Childlessness in the 1970s." *Journal of Marriage and the Family* 41:245–257.

Blumer, H. 1969. *Symbolic Interaction: Perspective and Method*. Englewood Cliffs, N.J.: Prentice-Hall.

Blumstein, P., and P. Schwartz. 1983. *American Couples: Money, Work, Sex*. New York: William Morrow.

Bohannan, P., and L. Bohannan. 1969. *A Source Notebook on Tiv Religion*. 5 vols. New Haven: HRAF.

Borkman, T. 1984. "Mutual Self-Help Groups: Strengthening the Selectively Unsupportive Personal and Community Networks of Their Members." In *The Self-Help Revolution*, ed. A. Gartner and F. Pressman, 205–215. New York: Human Sciences Press.

Brody, L. R. 1985. "Gender Differences in Emotional Development: A Review of Theories and Research." *Journal of Personality* 53:102–149.

Brown, J. B. 1986. "Gonadotropins." In *Infertility: Male and Female*, ed. V. Insler and B. Lunenfeld, 359–396. Edinburgh: Churchill Livingstone.

Buchman, M. 1989. *The Script of Life in Modern Society*. Chicago: University of Chicago Press.

Buechler, H. C., and J. Buechler. 1971. *The Bolivian Aymara*. New York: Holt, Rinehart, and Winston.

Bullock, J. C. 1974. "Iatrogenic Impotence in an Infertility Clinic: An Illustrative Case." *American Journal of Obstetrics and Gynecology* 12:476–478.

Bulman, R. J., and C. B. Wortman. 1977. "Attributions of Blame and Coping in the 'Real World': Severe Accident Victims React to Their Lot." *Journal of Personality and Social Psychology* 35:351–363.

Burgoyne, J. 1987. "Change, Gender, and the Lifecourse." In *Social Change and the Lifecourse*, ed. G. Cohen, 33–66. London: Tavistock.

Burgwyn, D. 1981. *Marriage Without Children*. New York: Harper & Row.

Bury, M. 1982. "Chronic Illness as Biographic Disruption." *Sociology of Health and Illness* 4:167–182.

Busfield, J. 1987. "Parenting and Parenthood." In *Social Change and the Life Course*, ed. G. Cohen, 67–86. London: Tavistock.

Busfield, J., and M. Paddon. 1977. *Thinking about Children*. London: Cambridge University Press.

Calame-Griaule, G. 1986. *Words and the Dogon World*. Philadelphia: Institute for Human Issues.

Caldwell, R., and L. Peplau. 1982. "Sex Differences in Same-Sex Friendship." *Sex Roles* 8:721–732.

Callan, V. J. 1983. "Perceptions of Parenthood and Childlessness: A Comparison of Mothers and Voluntarily Childless Wives." *Population and Environment* 6:179–189.

―――. 1987. "The Personal and Marital Adjustment of Mothers and of Voluntarily and Involuntarily Childless Wives." *Journal of Marriage and the Family* 49:847–856.

Cancian, F. M. 1987. *Love in America: Gender and Self-Development*. Cambridge: Cambridge University Press.

Cancian, F. M., and S. L. Gordon. 1988. "Changing Emotion Norms in Marriage: Love and Anger in U.S. Women's Magazines since 1900." *Gender & Society* 2:308–342.

Carlson, J. 1976. "The Sexual Role." In *Role Structure and Analysis of the Family*, ed. F. I. Nye, 101–110. Beverly Hills, Calif.: Sage.

Chaiklin, H., and M. Warfield. 1977. "Stigma Management and Amputee Rehabilitation." In *Social and Psychological Aspects of Disability*, ed. J. Stebbins, 103–111. Baltimore: University Park Press.

Charmaz, K. 1983. "Loss of Self: A Fundamental Form of Suffering in the Chronically Ill." *Sociology of Health and Illness* 5:168–195.

―――. 1987. "Struggling for a Self: Identity Levels of the Chronically Ill." *Research in the Sociology of Health Care* 6:283–321.

Christensen, J. B. 1954. *Double Descent Among the Fanti*. New Haven: HRAF.

Clarke, A. 1988. "The Industrialization of Human Reproduction, c. 1890–1990." Plenary address of annual conference of the University of California System-wide Council of Women's Programs. Davis, California, April 9.

Collier, J. F., and M. Z. Rosaldo. 1981. "Politics and Gender in Simple Societies." In *Sexual Meanings: The Cultural Construction of Gender and Sexuality*, ed. S. B. Ortner and H. Whitehead, 275–330. Cambridge: Cambridge University Press.

Collins, J. A., W. Wrixon, L. B. Janes, and E. H. Wilson. 1983. "Treatment-Independent Pregnancy Among Infertile Couples." *New England Journal of Medicine* 309:1201–1206.

Collins, J. A., J. B. Garner, E. W. Wilson, W. Wrixon, and R. F. Casper. 1984. "A Proportional Hazards Analysis of the Clinical Characteristics of Infertile Couples." *American Journal of Obstetrics and Gynecology* 148:527–532.

Collins, R. 1979. *The Credential Society*. New York: Academic Press.

Comaroff, J., and R. Maguire. 1986. "Ambiguity and the Search for Meaning: Childhood Leukemia in the Modern Clinical Context." In *The Sociology of Health and Illness: Critical Perspectives*, ed. P. Conrad and R. Kern, 100–109. 2d ed. New York: St. Martins.

Connolly, K. J., R. J. Edelmann, and I. D. Cooke. 1987. "Distress and Marital

Problems Associated with Infertility." *Journal of Reproductive and Infant Psychology* 5:49–57.

Conrad, P. 1985. "The Meaning of Medications: Another Look at Compliance." *Social Science and Medicine* 20:29–37.

———. 1987. "The Experience of Illness: Recent and New Directions." *Research in the Sociology of Health Care* 6:1–31.

Conrad, P., and R. Kern, eds. 1986. *The Sociology of Health and Illness: Critical Perspectives*. New York: St. Martins.

Conrad, P., and J. W. Schneider. 1980a. *Deviance and Medicalization: From Badness to Sickness*. St. Louis: Mosby.

———. 1980b. "Looking at Levels of Medicalization: A Comment on Strong's Critique of the Thesis of Medical Imperialism." *Social Science and Medicine* 14A:75–79.

Cook, E. P. 1987. "Characteristics of the Biosocial Crisis of Infertility." *Journal of Counseling and Development* 65:465–470.

Cook, J. A., and D. W. Wimberly. 1983. "If I Should Die Before I Wake: Religious Commitment and Adjustment to the Death of a Child." *Journal for the Scientific Study of Religion* 22:222–238.

Corea, G. 1977. *The Hidden Malpractice: How American Medicine Treats Women as Patients and Professionals*. New York: Morrow.

———. 1985. *The Mother Machine: Reproductive Technologies from Artificial Insemination to Artificial Wombs*. New York: Harper & Row.

Corea, G., R. D. Klein, L. Hanmer, H. B. Holmes, B. Hoskins, M. Kishwar, J. Raymond, R. Rowland, and R. Steinbacher. 1987. *Man-Made Women: How New Reproductive Technologies Affect Women*. Bloomington: Indiana University Press.

Cott, N. F. 1977. *The Bonds of Womanhood*. New Haven: Yale University Press.

Cozby, P. C. 1973. "Self-Disclosure: A Literature Review." *Psychological Bulletin* 79:73–91.

Crawford, R. 1986. "Individual Responsibility and Health Politics." In *The Sociology of Health and Illness: Critical Perspectives*, ed. P. Conrad and R. Kern, 369–377. 2d ed. New York: St. Martin's.

Crowe, C. 1985. "'Women Want It': *In Vitro* Fertilization and Women's Motivations for Participation." *Women's Studies International Forum* 8:57–62.

Cypress, B. K. 1984. "Patterns of Ambulatory Care in Obstetrics and Gynecology: The National Ambulatory Medical Care Survey, United States, January 1980–December 1981." Data from the National Health Survey, Series 13, no. 76.

Daly, K. 1988. "Reshaped Parenthood Identity: The Transition to Adoptive Parenthood." *Journal of Contemporary Ethnography* 17:40–66.

Daniels, A. K. 1987. "Invisible Work." *Social Problems* 34:403–415.

Daniluk, J. C., A. Leader, and P. L. Taylor. 1987. "Psychological and Relationship

Changes of Couples Undergoing an Infertility Investigation: Some Implications for Counseling." *British Journal of Guidance and Counseling* 15:29–36.

Danziger, S. K. 1986. "The Uses of Expertise in Doctor-Patient Encounters During Pregnancy." In *The Sociology of Health and Illness: Critical Perspectives*, ed. P. Conrad and R. Kern, 310–321. 2d ed. New York: St. Martins.

Davajan, V., and D. R. Mishell, Jr. 1986. "Evaluation of the Infertile Couple." In *Infertility, Contraception, and Reproductive Endocrinology*, ed. D. R. Mishell, Jr., and V. Davajan, 381–387. Oradell, N.J.: Medical Economics Books.

Davidson, J., and L. Duberman. 1982. "Same-Sex Friendships: A Gender Comparison of Dyads." *Sex Roles* 8:809–822.

Davis, F. 1961. "Deviance Disavowal: The Management of Strained Interaction by the Visibly Handicapped." *Social Problems* 9:120–132.

Davis, K., and D. Rowland. 1987. "Uninsured and Underserved: Inequities in Health Care in the United States." In *Dominant Issues in Medical Sociology*, ed. H. Schwartz, 511–526. 2d ed. New York: Random House.

Debrovner, C. H., and R. Shubin-Stein. 1976. "Sexual Problems Associated with Infertility." *Medical Aspects of Human Sexuality* 10:161–162.

Degler, C. 1980. *At Odds: Women and the Family in America from the Revolution to the Present*. New York: Oxford University Press.

DeJong, G. F., G. T. Cornwall, S. L. Hanson, and C. S. Stokes. 1984. "Childless and One-child, But Not by Choice: A Note on the Long-term Consequences for Life Satisfaction of Rural-reared Married Women." *Rural Sociology* 49:441–451.

Demos, J. 1986. *Past, Present, and Personal: The Family and the Life Course in American History*. New York: Oxford University Press.

Dennerstein, L., and C. Morse. 1988. "A Review of Psychological and Social Aspects of *In Vitro* Fertilization." *Journal of Psychosomatic Obstetrics and Gynecology* 9:159–170.

Dieterlen, G. 1941. *Les ames des Dogons*. Paris: Université, Institute d'Ethnologie, Travaux et Memoires 40.

Donchin, A. 1986. "The Future of Mothering: Reproductive Technology and Feminist Theory." *Hypatia* 1:121–137.

Dor, J., R. Hamber, and E. Rabau. 1977. "An Evaluation of Etiologic Factors and Therapy in 665 Infertile Couples." *Fertility and Sterility* 28:718–722.

Dorsey, G. A., and J. R. Murie. 1940. "Notes on Skidi Pawnee Society." *Field Museum of Natural History Anthropology Series* 27(2):65–119.

Dosch, A. 1910. "Not Enough Babies to Go Around." *Cosmopolitan*, Sept., 431–439.

Dougherty, C. J. 1988. *American Health Care: Realities, Rights, and Reforms*. New York: Oxford University Press.

Dworkin, A. 1983. *Right-Wing Women*. New York: Perigee Books.

Ebin, V. 1982. "Interpretations of Infertility: The Aowin People of Southwest Ghana." In *Ethnography of Fertility and Birth*, ed. C. P. MacCormack, 141–159. London: Academic Press.

Ehrenreich, B., and J. Ehrenreich. 1970. *The American Health Empire: Power, Profits, and Politics*. New York: Random House.

Ehrenreich, B., and D. English. 1979. *For Her Own Good: 150 Years of the Experts' Advice to Women*. Garden City, N.Y.: Anchor.

Engel, G. L. 1977. "The Need for a New Medical Model: A Challenge for Bio-medicine." *Science* 196(April 8):129–136.

Erlich, V. S. 1966. *Family in Transition: A Study of 300 Yugoslav Villages*. Princeton: Princeton University Press.

Falwell, J. 1987. "God's Way Is Still the Best Way." *USA Today*, March 18, 6A.

Feinberg, R. 1984. "Finding Homes for Children: The Process and the Literature." *Reference Services Review* 12:43–48.

Fenton, J., and A. Lifchez. 1980. *The Fertility Handbook*. New York: Clarkson, Potter.

FerreFax. 1990. "Bill Would Aid Infertility, Birth Control Research." *FerreFax* 6(1):5.

Field, M. J. 1970. *Search for Security: An Ethno Psychiatric Study of Rural Ghana*. New York: Norton.

Fife, A. E., and A. S. Fife. 1966. *Saints of Sage and Saddle: Folklore Among the Mormons*. Gloucester, Mass.: Peter Smith.

Firth, R. 1940. *The Work of the Gods in Tikopia*. Monographs on Social Anthropology, nos. 1 and 2. London: London School of Economics and Political Science.

Fischer, A. 1963. "Reproduction in Truk." *Ethnology* 2:526–540.

Fisher, S. 1988. *In the Patient's Best Interest: Women and the Politics of Medical Decisions*. New Brunswick, N.J.: Rutgers University Press.

Fisher, S., and A. D. Todd. 1983. *The Social Organization of Doctor-Patient Communication*. Washington: Center for Applied Linguistics.

Fitzpatrick, M. A., and J. Indvik. 1982. "The Instrumental and Expressive Domains of Marital Communication." *Human Communication Research* 8:195–213.

Flemming, J. 1984. "Infertility as a Chronic Illness." *Resolve Newsletter*, Dec., 5.

Ford, C. 1945. *A Comparative Study of Human Reproduction*. New Haven: Yale University Publications in Anthropology.

Fox, C. E. 1966. "Pregnancy, Childbirth, and Early Infancy in Anglo-American Culture: 1675–1830." Ph.D. diss., University of Pennsylvania.

Francis, V., B. M. Korsch, and M. J. Morris. 1969. "Gaps in Doctor-Patient Communication." *New England Journal of Medicine* 280:535–540.

Frank, E. C., Anderson, and D. Rubinstein. 1979. "Marital Role Strain and Sexual Satisfaction." *Journal of Consulting and Clinical Psychology* 47:1096–1103.

Franklin, S., and M. McNeil. 1988. "Reproductive Futures: Recent Literature and Current Debates on Reproductive Technologies." *Feminist Studies* 14:545–560.

Freeman, E. W., A. S. Boxer, K. Rickels, R. Tureck, and L. Mastroianni, Jr. 1985. "Psychological Evaluation and Support in a Program of *In Vitro* Fertilization and Embryo Transfer." *Fertility and Sterility* 4:48–53.

Freeman, J. D. 1955. *Iban Agriculture: A Report on the Shifting Cultivation of Hill Rice by the Iban of Sarawak.* Colonial Research Studies, no. 18. London: H. M. Stationery Office.

Friedson, E. 1966. "Disability as Social Deviance." In *Sociology and Rehabilitation*, ed. M. Sussman, 71–99. Washington: American Sociological Association.

―――. 1970. *Profession of Medicine: A Study in the Sociology of Applied Knowledge.* New York: Dodd, Mead.

Fry, C. L. 1983. "Temporal and Status Dimensions of Life Cycles." *International Journal of Aging and Human Development* 17:281–300.

Galaal, M. H. I. 1968. *The Terminology and Practice of Somali Weather, Astronomy and Astrology.* Mogadishu: Self-published.

Gartner, A., and F. Riessman, eds. 1984. *The Self-Help Revolution.* New York: Human Sciences Press.

Gebhard, B. 1976. "The Interrelationship of Scientific and Folk Medicine in the United States of America since 1850." In *American Folk Medicine: A Symposium*, ed. W. D. Hand, 87–97. Berkeley: University of California Press.

Gebhard, P. 1966. "Factors in Marital Orgasm." *Journal of Social Issues* 22:88–95.

Geertz, C. 1968. "Religion as a Cultural System." In *Anthropological Approaches to the Study of Religion*, ed. M. Banton, 1–46. London: Tavistock.

Gladwin, T., and S. B. Sarason. 1953. *Truk: Man in Paradise.* Viking Fund Publications in Anthropology, no. 20. New York: Wenner-Gren Foundation for Anthropological Research.

Glassner, B. 1988. *Bodies: Why We Look The Way We Do (and How We Feel About It).* New York: Putnam's.

Goffman, E. 1963. *Stigma: Notes on the Management of Spoiled Identity.* Englewood Cliffs, N.J.: Prentice-Hall.

Golden, G. H. 1983. "Psychosexual Problems in Infertility: A Preventive Model." *Journal of Sex Education and Therapy* 9:19–22.

Gomel, V., P. J. Taylor, A. A. Yuzpe, and J. E. Rioux. 1986. *Laparoscopy and Hysteroscopy in Gynecologic Practice.* Chicago: Year Book Medical Publishers.

Gonzalez, M. L., and D. W. Emmons. 1988. *Socioeconomic Characteristics of Medical Practice, 1988.* Chicago: American Medical Association.

Goody, J. 1976. *Production and Reproduction.* Cambridge: Cambridge University Press.

Gormly, A. V., J. B. Gormly, and H. Weiss. 1987. "Motivations for Parenthood Among Young Adult College Students." *Sex Roles* 16:31–39.

References

Grabill, W. H., C. Kiser, and P. Whelpton. 1973. "A Long View." In *The American Family in Social-Historical Perspective*, ed. M. Gordon, 374–396. New York: St. Martin's.

Graham, S., and L. G. Reeder. 1979. "Social Epidemiology of Chronic Diseases." In *Handbook of Medical Sociology*, ed. H. E. Freeman, S. Levine, and L. G. Reeder, 71–96. 3d ed. Englewood Cliffs, N.J.: Prentice-Hall.

Gramling, R., and C. J. Forsyth. 1987. "Exploiting Stigma." *Sociological Forum* 2:401–415.

Greeley, A. M. 1972. *The Denominational Society: A Sociological Approach to Religion in America*. Glenview, Ill.: Scott, Foresman.

Greenblat, C. S. 1983. "The Salience of Sexuality in the Early Years of Marriage." *Journal of Marriage and The Family* 45:289–299.

Greer, G. 1984. *Sex and Destiny: The Politics of Human Fertility*. New York: Harper & Row.

Greil, A. L. 1989. "The Technology of Reproduction: Religious Responses." *The Christian Century* 106:11–14.

Greil, A. L., and T. A. Leitko. 1985. "Religiosity and Well-being among Infertile Couples." Paper presented at the annual meeting, Association for the Sociology of Religion. Washington, D.C.

Greil, A., T. A. Leitko, and K. L. Porter. 1988. "Infertility: His and Hers." *Gender and Society* 2:172–199.

———. 1989. "Sex and Intimacy Among Infertile Couples." *Journal of Psychology and Human Sexuality* 2:117–138.

Greil, A., and K. L. Porter. 1988. "Explaining Treatment Addiction Among Infertile Couples." Paper presented at the annual meeting, National Council of Family Relations. Philadelphia, Pa.

Greil, A. L., K. L. Porter, T. A. Leitko, and C. Riscilli. 1989. "Why Me?: Theodicies of Infertile Women and Men." *Sociology of Health and Illness* 11:213–229.

Griffis, W. E. 1882. *Corea: The Hermit Nation*. New York: Scribner's.

Gruhn, J. G., and R. R. Kazer. 1989. *Hormonal Regulation of the Menstrual Cycle: Evolution of Concepts*. New York: Plenum Medical Book Co.

Gurdon, P. R. T. 1907. *The Khasis*. London: David Nutt.

Gussow, Z., and G. S. Tracy. 1968. "Status, Ideology and Adaptation to Stigmatized Illness: A Study of Leprosy." *Human Organization* 27:316–325.

Halle, D. 1984. *America's Working Man: Work, Home, and Politics Among Blue-Collar Property Owners*. Chicago: University of Chicago Press.

Hanks, M., and D. E. Poplin. 1981. "The Sociology of Physical Disability: A Review of the Literature and Some Conceptual Perspectives." *Deviant Behavior* 2:309–328.

Hanson, S. L., G. T. Cornwall, G. F. DeJong, and C. S. Stokes. 1984. "Consequences of Involuntary Low Parity for Women's Perceptions of Homemaker and Work Roles: Findings from a 24-year Longitudinal Study." *Social Science Research* 68:327–349.

Hareven, T. 1977. "Family Time and Historical Time." *Daedalus* 106:57–70.

———. 1984. "Themes in the Historical Development of the Family." In *Review of Child Development Research*, Vol. 7: *The Family*, ed. R. D. Parke, 137–178. Chicago: University of Chicago Press.

Harris, S. 1950. *Women's Surgeon: The Life Story of J. Marian Sims*. New York: Macmillan.

Haseltine, F. P., C. Mazure, W. De L'Aune, D. Greenfeld, N. Laufer, B. Tarlatzis, M. L. Polan, E. E. Jones, R. Graebe, F. Nero, A. D'Lugi, D. Fazio, J. Masters, and A. H. DeCherney. 1985. "Psychological Interviews in Screening Couples Undergoing *In Vitro* Fertilization." *Annals of the New York Academy of Sciences* 442:504–522.

Hayes-Bautista, D. E. 1976. "Modifying the Treatment: Patient Compliance, Patient Control and Medical Care." *Social Science and Medicine* 10:233–238.

Heer, D. M. 1962. "Husband and Wife Perceptions of Family Power Structure." *Marriage and Family Living* 24:56–57.

Hendershot, G. E. 1984. "Maternal Age and Overdue Conceptions." American *Journal of Public Health* 74:35–37.

Herzlich, C., and J. Pierret. 1987. *Illness and Self in Society*. Baltimore: Johns Hopkins University Press.

Hilbert, A. 1984. "The Cultural Dimensions of Chronic Pain: Flawed Reality Construction and the Problem of Meaning." *Social Problems* 31:365–378.

Hilger, M. I. 1951. "Chippewa Child Life and Its Cultural Background." *Bureau of American Ethnology Bulletin* 146. Washington: Smithsonian Institution.

Hirsch, M. B., and W. D. Mosher. 1987. "Characteristics of Infertile Women in the United States and Their Use of Fertility Services." *Fertility and Sterility* 47:618–625.

Hochschild, A. R. 1983. *The Managed Heart: Commercialization of Human Feeling*. Berkeley: University of California Press.

———. 1989. *The Second Shift: Working Parents and the Revolution at Home*. New York: Viking.

Hoffman, L. W., and J. D. Manis. 1979. "The Value of Children in the United States: A New Approach to the Study of Fertility." *Journal of Marriage and the Family* 41:583–596.

Hogan, D. P., and N. M. Astone. 1986. "The Transition to Adulthood." *Annual Review of Sociology* 12:109–130.

Holman, J. F., and C. B. Hammond. 1988. "Induction of Ovulation with Clomiphene Citrate." In *Progress in Infertility*, ed. S. J. Behrman, R. W. Kistner, and G. W. Patton, 499–511. Boston: Little, Brown.

References

Houseknecht, S. H. 1979. "Childlessness and Marital Adjustment." *Journal of Marriage and the Family* 41:259–265.

————. 1987. "Voluntary Childlessness." In *Handbook of Marriage and the Family*, ed. M. B. Sussman and S. K. Steinmetz, 369–395. New York: Plenum.

Hubbard, R. 1981. "The Case Against *In Vitro* Fertilization and Implantation." In *The Custom-made Child*, ed. H. Holmes, B. B. Hoskins, and M. Gross, 159–162. Clifton, N.J.: Humana Press.

Hughes, E. C. 1945. "Dilemmas and Contradictions in Status." *American Journal of Sociology* 50:353–359.

Hull, M. G. K., C. M. A. Glazener, N. J. Kelly, D. I. Conway, P. A. Foster, R. A. Hinton, C. Coulson, P. A. Lambert, E. M. Watt, and K. M. Desai. 1985. "Population Study of Causes, Treatment and Outcome of Infertility." *British Medical Journal* 291:1693–1697.

Hunt, M. 1970. *Sexual Behavior in the Seventies*. Chicago: Playboy.

Huston, T. L., and R. D. Ashmore. 1986. "Women and Men in Personal Relationships." In *The Social Psychology of Female-Male Relations: A Critical Analysis of Central Concepts*, ed. R. D. Ashmore and F. K. DelBoca, 167–210. New York: Academic Press.

Illich, I. 1976. *Medical Nemesis: The Expropriation of Health*. New York: Pantheon.

Insler, V., G. Potashnik, and M. Glassner. 1981. "Some Epidemiological Aspects of Fertility Evaluation." In *Advances in Diagnosis and Treatment of Infertility*, ed. V. Insler and G. Bettendorf, 165–177. New York: Elsevier/North-Holland.

Jamison, P. H., L. R. Fanzini, and R. M. Kaplan. 1979. "Some Assumed Characteristics of Voluntarily Childfree Women and Men." *Psychology of Women Quarterly* 4:266–273.

Jones, L. F. 1944. *A Study of the Tlingets of Alaska*. New York: Fleming H. Revell.

Kalmuss, D. S. 1987. "The Use of Infertility Services among Fertility-impaired Couples." *Demography* 24:575–585.

Kandiyoti, D. 1988. "Bargaining with Patriarchy." *Gender & Society* 2:274–290.

Kass, L. R. 1971. "Babies by Means of *In Vitro* Fertilization: Unethical Experiments on the Unborn?" *New England Journal of Medicine* 285:1174–1179.

Katayama, K. P., K. Ju, M. Manuel, G. S. Jones, and H. W. Jones, Jr. 1979. "Computer Analysis of Etiology and Pregnancy Rate in 636 Cases of Infertility." *American Journal of Obstetrics and Gynecology* 135:207–214.

Katz, S. S., and S. H. Katz. 1987. "An Evaluation of Traditional Therapy for Barrenness." *Medical Anthropology Quarterly* 1:394–405.

Kaufman, D. R. 1985. "Women Who Return to Orthodox Judaism: A Feminist Analysis." *Journal of Marriage and the Family* 47:543–551.

Kaufman, S. A. 1969. "Impact of Infertility on the Marital and Sexual Relationship." *Fertility and Sterility* 20:380–383.

Kelley, D. M. 1977. *Why Conservative Churches are Growing*. San Francisco: Harper & Row.

Kemeter, P., A. Eder, and M. Springer-Kremser. 1985. "Psychosocial Testing and Pretreatment of Women for *In Vitro* Fertilization." *Annals of the New York Academy of Sciences* 442:523–532.

Kitagawa, E. M., and P. M. Hauser. 1973. *Differential Mortality in the United States: A Study in Social Epidemiology*. Cambridge: Cambridge University Press.

Klagsbrun, F. 1985. *Married People: Staying Together in the Age of Divorce*. Toronto: Bantam.

Kleinman, A. 1988. *The Illness Narratives: Suffering, Healing, and the Human Condition*. New York: Basic.

Kliger, B. E. 1984. "Evaluation, Therapy, and Outcome in 493 Infertile Couples." *Fertility and Sterility* 41:40–46.

Knaub, P. K., D. B. Eversoll, and J. H. Voss. 1983. "Is Parenthood a Desired Role?: An Assessment Of Attitudes Held by Contemporary Women." *Sex Roles* 9:355–362.

Knowles, J. H. 1977. "The Responsibility of the Individual." In *Doing Better and Feeling Worse: Health in the United States*, ed. John H. Knowles, 57–80. New York: Norton.

Kohli, M. 1986. "The World We Forgot: A Historical Review of the Life Course." In *Later Life: The Social Psychology of Aging*, ed. V. W. Marshall, 271–303. Beverly Hills: Sage.

Komarovsky, M. 1962. *Blue-Collar Marriage*. New York: Vintage.

———. 1974. "Patterns of Self-Disclosure of Male Undergraduates." *Journal of Marriage and the Family* 36:677–686.

Korsch, B. M., and V. F. Negrete. 1972. "Doctor-Patient Communication." *Scientific American*, Aug., 66–74.

Kotarba, J. A. 1983. "Perception of Death, Belief Systems, and the Process of Coping with Chronic Pain." *Social Science and Medicine* 17:681–689.

Kraft, A. D., J. Palombro, D. Mitchell, C. Dean, S. Meyers, and A. W. Schmidt. 1980. "The Psychological Dimensions of Infertility." *American Journal of Orthopsychiatry* 50:618–627.

Krokoff, K. J. 1987. "The Correlates of Negative Affect in Marriage: An Exploratory Study of Gender Differences." *Journal of Family Issues* 8:111–135.

Kroll-Smith, J. S., and S. R. Couch. 1987. "A Chronic Technical Disaster and the Irrelevance of Religious Meaning: The Case of Centralia, Pennsylvania." *Journal for the Scientific Study of Religion* 26:25–37.

Kushner, H. S. 1981. *When Bad Things Happen to Good People*. New York: Schocken.

Ladd-Taylor, M. 1986. *Raising a Baby the Government Way: Mothers' Letters to the Children's Bureau, 1915–1932*. New Brunswick, N.J.: Rutgers University Press.

Lalos, A., O. Lalos, L. Jacobsson, and B. von Schoultz. 1985. "The Psychosocial Impact of Infertility Two Years After Completed Surgical Treatment." *Acta Obstetrica et Gynecologica Scandinavia* 64:599–604.

Lasch, C. 1977. *Haven in a Heartless World*. New York: Basic.

Lasker, J. N. 1988. "Women, Men and Reproductive Technology." Paper presented at the annual meeting of the Society for the Study of Social Problems, August, Atlanta.

Lasker, J. N., and S. Borg. 1987. *In Search of Parenthood: Coping with Infertility and High-Tech Conception*. Boston: Beacon.

Lauritzen, P. 1990. "What Price Parenthood?" *Hastings Center Report* 20(2):38–47.

Leavitt, J. W. 1986. *Brought to Bed: Childbearing in America, 1750 to 1950*. New York: Oxford University Press.

Lee, D. D. 1953. "Copulou, Greece." In *Cultural Patterns and Technical Change*, ed. M. Mead, 77–114. Paris: UNESCO.

Leerhsen, C. 1990. "Unite and Conquer." *Newsweek*, Feb. 5, 50–55.

Lehman, D. R., C. B. Wortman, and A. F. Williams. 1987. "Long-term Effects of Losing a Spouse or Child in a Motor Vehicle Crash." *Journal of Personality and Social Psychology* 52:218–231.

Leitko, T. A., and A. L. Greil. 1985. "Gender, Involuntary Childlessness, and Emotional Distress." Paper presented at the annual meeting of the American Sociological Association. Washington, D.C.

Lerner, M. 1980. *The Belief in a Just World*. New York: Plenum.

Levitin, T. E. 1979. "Deviants as Active Participants in the Labeling Process: The Visibly Handicapped." In *Health, Illness, and Medicine*, ed. G. L. Albrecht and P. C. Higgins, 217–227. Chicago: Rand McNally.

Lewis, J. S. 1986. *In the Family Way: Childbearing in the British Aristocracy, 1760–1860*. New Brunswick, N.J.: Rutgers University Press.

Link, P. W., and C. A. Darling. 1986. "Couples Undergoing Treatment for Infertility: Dimensions of Life Satisfaction." *Journal of Sex and Marital Therapy* 12:46–59.

Lorber, J. 1967. "Deviance as Performance: The Case of Illness." *Social Problems* 14:302–310.

———. 1988. "Gender Politics and *In Vitro* Fertilization Use." In *Embryos, Ethics, and Women's Rights: Exploring the New Reproductive Technologies*, ed. E. H. Baruch, A. F. D'Adamio, Jr., and J. Seager, 117–133. New York: Harrington Park Press.

———. 1989. "Choice, Gift, or Patriarchal Bargain?: Women's Consent to *In Vitro* Fertilization in Male Infertility." *Hypatia* 4:23–36.

Lorber, J., and D. Greenfield, 1989. "Couple's Experiences with *In Vitro* Fertilization: A Phenomenological Approach." Paper presented at Sixth World Congress on IVF and Assisted Reproduction, April, Jerusalem.

References

Luckmann, T. 1967. *The Invisible Religion*. New York: Macmillan.

Lynd, R. S., and H. M. Lynd. 1929. *Middletown: A Study in Contemporary American Culture*. New York: Harcourt Brace.

———. 1982. *Middletown in Transition: A Study in Culture Conflicts*. New York: Harcourt Brace Jovanovich.

Macomber, D. 1924. "Prevention of Sterility." *Journal of the American Medical Association* 83:678–682.

Mahlstedt, P. 1985. "The Psychological Component of Infertility." *Fertility and Sterility* 43:335–346.

Mahlstedt, P., S. MacDuff, and J. Bernstein. 1987. "Emotional Factors and the *In Vitro* Fertilization and Embryo Transfer Process." *Journal of In Vitro Fertilization and Embryo Transfer* 4:232–236.

Mair, L. P. 1934. *An African People in the Twentieth Century*. London: Routledge.

Markman, H. 1984. "The Longitudinal Study of Couples' Interactions: Implications for Understanding and Predicting the Development of Marital Stress." In *Marital Interaction: Analysis and Modification*, ed. K. Hahlweg and N. Jacobsen, 253–281. New York: Guilford.

Martin, E. 1987. *The Woman in the Body: A Cultural Analysis of Reproduction*. Boston: Beacon.

Martin Matthews, A., and R. Matthews. 1986. "Beyond the Mechanics of Infertility: Perspectives on the Social Psychology of Infertility and Involuntary Childlessness." *Family Relations* 35:479–487.

Masters, W. M. 1953. *Rowanduz: A Kurdish Administrative and Mercantile Center*. Ph.D. diss., University of Michigan.

Mattesich, P. W. 1979. "Childlessness and its Correlates in Historical Perspective: A Research Note." *Journal of Family History* 4:299–307.

Matthews, R., and A. Martin Matthews. 1986. "Infertility and Involuntary Childlessness: The Transition to Nonparenthood." *Journal of Marriage and the Family* 48:641–649.

Mazor, M. D. 1979. "Barren Couples." *Psychology Today* May, 101–112.

———. 1980. "Psychosexual Problems of the Infertile Couple." *Medical Aspects of Human Sexuality* 14:32–49.

———. 1984. "Emotional Reactions to Infertility." In *Infertility: Medical, Emotional, and Social Considerations*, ed. M. D. Mazor and H. F. Simons, 23–35. New York: Human Sciences Press.

McCormick, T. 1980. "Out of Control: One Aspect of Infertility." *Journal of Obstetrical, Gynecological and Neonatal Nursing* 9:205–206.

McEwan, K. L., C. G. Costello, and P. J. Taylor. 1987. "Adjustment to Infertility." *Abnormal Psychology* 96:108–116.

McGregor, D. K. 1986. "Silver Sutures: The Medical Career of J. Marion Sims." Ph.D. diss., State University of New York at Binghamton.

References

McGuire, M. B. 1981. *Religion: The Social Context*. Belmont, Calif.: Wadsworth.

————, with the assistance of D. Kantor. 1988. *Ritual Healing in Suburban America*. New Brunswick, N.J.: Rutgers University Press.

McLane, C. M., and M. McLane. 1969. "A Half Century of Sterility 1840–1890." *Fertility and Sterility* 20:853–870.

Mechanic, D. 1968. *Medical Sociology*. Glencoe, Ill.: Free Press.

Medical Research International and the Society of Assisted Reproductive Technology. 1989. "*In Vitro* Fertilization/Embryo Transfer in the United States: 1987 Results from the National IVF-ET Registry." *Fertility and Sterility* 51:13–19.

Menning, B. E. 1977. *Infertility: A Guide for Childless Couples*. Englewood Cliffs, N.J.: Prentice-Hall.

————. 1979. "Counselling Infertile Couples." *Contemporary Obstetrics and Gynecology* 13:101–108.

————. 1982. "The Psychological Impact of Infertility." *Nursing Clinics of North America* 17:155–163.

Messing, S. D. 1957. "The Highland Plateau Amhara of Ethiopia." Ph.D. diss., University of Pennsylvania.

Miall, C. E. 1985. "Perceptions of Informal Sanctioning and the Stigma of Involuntary Childlessness." *Deviant Behavior* 6:383–403.

————. 1986. "The Stigma of Involuntary Childlessness." *Social Problems* 33:268–282.

————. 1987. "The Stigma of Adoptive Parent Status: Perceptions of Community Attitudes toward Adoption and the Experience of Informal Social Sanctioning." *Family Relations* 36:34–39.

Mishler, E. G. 1984. *The Discourse of Medicine*. Norwood, N.J.: Ablex.

Mishler, E. G., L. R. AmaraSingham, S. D. Osherson, S. T. Hauser, N. E. Waxler, and F. Liem. 1981. *Social Contexts of Health, Illness, and Patient Care*. Cambridge: Cambridge University Press.

Mizrahi, T. 1986. *Getting Rid of Patients: Contradictions in the Socialization of Physicians*. New Brunswick, N.J.: Rutgers University Press.

Modell, J. 1980. "Normative Aspects of American Marriage Timing since World War II." *Journal of Family History* 5:7–32.

————. 1989. *Into One's Own: From Youth to Adulthood in the United States, 1920–1975*. Berkeley: University of California Press.

Monroe, P. A., J. L. Bokemeier, J. Kotchen, and H. McKean. 1985. "Spousal Response Consistency in Decision-making Research." *Journal of Marriage and the Family* 7:733–738.

Moose, J. R. 1911. *Village Life in Korea*. Nashville: M. E. Church.

Morgan, B. 1976. "Intimacy of Disclosure Topics and Sex Difference in Self-Disclosure." *Sex Roles* 2:161–165.

Mornell, P. 1979. *Passive Men, Wild Women*. New York: Ballantine.

Morse, C. A., and E. Van Hall. 1987. "Psychosocial Aspects of Infertility: A Review of Current Concepts." *Journal of Psychosomatic Obstetrics and Gynecology* 6:157–164.

Mosher, W. D. 1982. "Infertility among U.S. Couples 1965–1976." *Family Planning Perspectives* 14:22–27.

———. 1987. "Infertility: Why Business is Booming." *American Demographics* 9:42–43.

Navarro, V. 1976. *Medicine Under Capitalism*. New York: Prodist.

Neugarten, B. L., J. W. Moore, and J. C. Lowe. 1965. "Age Norms, Age Constraints, and Adult Socialization." *American Journal of Sociology* 70:710–717.

Olshansky, E. F. 1987. "Identity of Self as Infertile: An Example of Theory-Generating Research." *Advances in Nursing Science* 9(2):54–63.

Origins. 1987. "Instruction on Respect for Human Life in Its Origins and on the Dignity of Procreation—Replies to Certain Questions of the Day." *Origins* 16:697–711.

Ory, M. 1978. "The Decision to Parent or Not: Normative and Structural Components." *Journal of Marriage and the Family* 40:531–539.

Osherson, S. D., and L. R. AmaraSingham. 1981. "The Machine Metaphor in Medicine." In *Social Contexts of Health, Illness, and Patient Care*, ed. G. Mishler, L. R. AmaraSingham, S. D. Osherson, S. T. Hauser, N. E. Waxler, and F. Liem, 218–259. Cambridge: Cambridge University Press.

Overall, C. 1987. *Ethics and Human Reproduction: A Feminist Analysis*. Boston: Allen and Unwin.

Owens, D. J., and M. W. Read. 1984. "Patients' Experience with and Assessment of Subfertility Testing and Treatment." *Journal of Reproductive and Infant Psychology* 2:7–17.

Page, H. 1989. "Estimation of the Prevalence and Incidence of Infertility in a Population: A Pilot Study." *Fertility and Sterility* 51:571–577.

Parelman, A. 1983. *Emotional Intimacy in Marriage: A Sex Roles Perspective*. Ann Arbor, Mich.: UMI Research Press.

Parin, P., F. Morgenthaler, and G. Parin-Matthes. 1963. *Die weissen denken zuviel: psychoanalytische untersuchungen bei den Dogon in Westafrika*. Zurich: Atlantis Verlag.

Parsons, T. 1958. "Definitions of Illness and Health in Light of American values and Social Structure." In *Patients, Physicians, and Illness*, ed. E. G. Jaco, 165–187. New York: Free Press.

Pasternak, B. 1972. *Kinship and Community in Two Chinese Villages*. Stanford: Stanford University Press.

References

Patton, D., and E. M. Waring. 1985. "Sex and Marital Intimacy." *Journal of Sex and Marital Therapy* 11:176–184.

Paulson, J. D., B. S. Haarmann, R. L. Salerno, and P. Asmar. 1988. "An Investigation of the Relationship between Emotional Maladjustment and Infertility." *Fertility and Sterility* 49:258–262.

Payer, L. 1988. *Medicine and Culture: Varieties of Treatment in the United States, England, West Germany, and France*. New York: Holt.

Pearsall, M. 1950. "Klamath Childhood and Education." *University of California Anthropological Records* 9:339–351.

Peplau, L., and S. Gordon. 1985. "Women and Men in Love: Sex Differences in Close Relationships." In *Women, Gender, and Social Psychology*, ed. V. O'Leary, R. Unger, and B. Wallston, 257–591. Hillsdale, N.Y.: Erlbaum.

Perlman, S. D., and P. R. Abramson. 1982. "Sexual Satisfaction among Married and Cohabitating Individuals." *Journal of Consulting and Clinical Psychology* 50:458–460.

Pern, S. 1982. *Masked Dancers of West Africa: The Dogon*. Amsterdam: Time-Life Books.

Pfeffer, N. 1987. "Artificial Insemination, *In Vitro* Fertilization, and the Stigma of Infertility." In *Reproductive Technologies: Gender, Motherhood, and Medicine*, ed. M. Stanworth, 81–97. Minneapolis: University of Minnesota Press.

Piker, S. I. 1975. "Changing Child-bearing practices in Central Thailand." *Contributions in Asian Studies* 8:90–108.

Pirie, M. 1988. "Women and the Illness Role: Rethinking Feminist Theory." *Canadian Review of Sociology and Anthropology* 25:628–648.

Plath, D., and K. Ikeda. 1976. "After Coming of Age: Adult Awareness of Age Norms." In *Socialization and Communication in Primary Groups*, ed. T. R. Williams, 107–123. The Hague: Morton.

Platt, J. J., Ficher and J. J. Silver. 1973. "Infertile Couples: Personality Traits and Self-Ideal Concept Discrepancies." *Fertility and Sterility* 24:972–976.

Plumez, J. H. 1980. "Adoption: Where Have All the Babies Gone?" *New York Times Magazine*, April 13, 34–42, 105–106.

Poole, E. D., R. M. Regoli, and M. R. Pogrebin. 1986. "A Study of the Effects of Self-Labelling and Public Labelling." *Social Sciences Journal* 23:345–360.

Pospisil, L. 1958. *Kapauku Papuans and Their Law*. Yale University Publications in Anthropology, no. 54. New Haven: Yale University Press.

Poston, D. L., K. B. Kramer, K. Trent, and M. Yu. 1983. "Estimating Voluntary and Involuntary Childlessness in Developing Countries." *Journal of Biosocial Science* 15:441–452.

Poston, D. L., and K. Trent. 1984. "Modernization and Childlessness in the Developing World." *Comparative Social Research* 7:133–153.

Preston, T. 1981. *Clay Pedestal*. Seattle: Madrona Publishers.

Radbill, S. X. 1976. "The Role of Animals in Infant Feeding." In *American Folk Medicine: A Symposium*, ed. W. D. Hand, 21–30. Berkeley: University of California Press.

Rainwater, L., R. P. Coleman, and G. Handel. 1959. *Workingman's Wife*. New York: ARNO Press.

Randle, M. C. 1951. "Iroquois Women: Then and Now." In *Symposium on Local Diversity in Iroquois Culture*, ed. W. N. Fenton, 167–187. Washington, D.C.: Smithsonian Institution.

Rattray, R. S. 1923. *Ashanti*. Oxford: Clarendon Press.

Raval, H., P. Slade, P. Buck, and B. E. Lieberman. 1987. "The Impact of Infertility on Emotions and the Marital and Sexual Relationship." *Journal of Reproductive and Infant Psychology* 5:221–234.

Raymont, A., G. H. Arronet, and W. S. M. Arrata. 1969. "Review of 500 Cases of Infertility". *International Journal of Fertility* 4:141–153.

Reed, K. 1987. "The Effect of Infertility on Female Sexuality." *Pre- and Peri-Natal Psychology Journal* 2:57–62.

Reinharz, S. 1988. "Controlling Women's Lives: A Cross-Cultural Interpretation of Miscarriage Accounts." *Research in the Sociology of Health Care* 7:3–37.

Reynolds, R. A., and R. L. Ohsfeldt. 1984. *Socioeconomic Characteristics of Medical Practice, 1984*. Chicago: Center for Health Policy Research.

Richards, A. 1956. *Chisungu: A Girl's Initiation Ceremony Among the Bemba of Northern Rhodesia*. London: Faber and Faber.

Ries, P. 1985. "Health Characteristics According to Family and Personal Income." U.S. Department of Health and Human Services, *Vital and Health Statistics*, series 10, no. 14. Washington, D.C.: U.S. Government Printing Office.

———. 1987. "Health Care Coverage by Age, Sex, Race, and Family Income: United States, 1986." U.S. Department of Health and Human Services, *Advance Data from Vital and Health Statistics*, no. 139. Washington, D.C.: U.S. Government Printing Office.

Riessman, C. K. 1974. "The Use of Health Services by the Poor." *Social Policy* 5:41–49.

———. 1983. "Women and Medicalization: A New Perspective." *Social Policy* 14:3–18.

———. 1990. *Divorce Talk: Women and Men Make Sense of Personal Relationships*. New Brunswick, N.J.: Rutgers University Press.

Rindfuss, R. R., L. L. Bumpass, and C. St. John. 1980. "Education and Fertility: Implications for the Roles Women Occupy." *American Sociological Review* 45:431–447.

Rindfuss, R. R., and C. St. John. 1983. "Social Determinants of Age at First Birth." *Journal of Marriage and the Family* 45:553–565.

References

Risman, B. 1987. "Intimate Relationships from a Microstructural Perspective: Mothering Men." *Gender & Society* 1:6–32.

Rohrer, J. H., and M. S. Edmonson. 1960. *The Eighth Generation: Cultures and Personalities of New Orleans Negroes*. New York: Harper.

Roscoe, J. 1911. *The Baganda: An Account of Their Native Customs and Beliefs*. London: Macmillan.

Rosenblatt, P. C., P. Peterson, J. Portner, M. Cleveland, A. Mykkanen, R. Foster, G. Holm, B. Joel, H. Reisch, C. Kreushcher, and R. Phillips. 1973. "A Cross-Cultural Study of Responses to Childlessness." *Behavior Science Notes* 8:221–231.

Ross, C. E., and R. S. Duff. 1983. "Medical Care, Living Conditions and Children's Well-being." *Social Forces* 61:456–474.

Roth, J. 1963. *Timetables*. Indianapolis: Bobbs-Merrill.

———. 1972. "Staff and Client Control Strategies in Urban Hospital Emergency Services." *Urban Life and Culture* 1:39–60.

Rothman, B. K. 1982. *In Labor: Women and Power in the Birthplace*. New York: Norton.

———. 1984. "The Meanings of Choice in Reproductive Technology." In *Test-Tube Women: What Future for Motherhood?* ed. R. Arditti, R. D. Klein, and S. Minden, 22–33. London: Pandora.

———. 1986. *The Tentative Pregnancy: Women's Experience with Amniocentesis*. New York: Viking.

———. 1989. *Recreating Motherhood: Ideology and Technology in a Patriarchal Society*. New York: Norton.

Rottenberg, M. 1975. "Self-Labeling Theory: Preliminary Findings among Mental Patients." *British Journal of Criminology* 15:360–375.

Rowland, R. 1987. "Technology and Motherhood: Reproductive Choice Reconsidered." *Signs: Journal of Women in Culture and Society* 12:512–518.

Rubin, L. B. 1976. *Worlds of Pain: Life in Working-Class Families*. New York: Basic.

———. 1983. *Intimate Strangers: Men and Women Together*. New York: Harper & Row.

Russo, N. F. 1976. "The Motherhood Mandate." *Journal of Social Issues* 32:143–151.

Ryder, N., and C. Westoff. 1971. *Reproduction in the United States: 1965*. Princeton, N.J.: Princeton University Press.

Sabatelli, R. M., R. L. Meth, and S. M. Gavazzi. 1988. "Factors Mediating the Adjustment to Involuntary Childlessness." *Family Relations* 37:338–343.

Sandelowski, M. 1987. "The Color Gray: Ambiguity and Infertility." *Image: Journal of Nursing Scholarship* 19:70–74.

———. 1988. "Without Child: The World of Infertile Women." *Health Care for Women International* 9:147–161.

_____. 1989. "Compelled to Try: The Problem of Persistence in the Treatment of Infertility." Manuscript.

_____. 1990. "Fault Lines: Infertility and Imperiled Sisterhood." *Feminist Studies* 16:33–51.

Sandelowski, M., and L. C. Jones. 1986. "Social Exchanges of Infertile Women." *Issues in Mental Health Nursing* 8:173–189.

Sandelowski, M., and C. Pollock. 1986. "Women's Experience of Infertility." *Image: Journal of Nursing Scholarship* 18:140–144.

Scambler, G. 1984. "Perceiving and Coping with a Stigmatizing Condition." In *The Experience of Illness*, ed. R. Fitzpatrick, J. Hinton, S. Newman, G. Scambler, and J. Thompson, 203–226. New York: Tavistock.

Scambler, G., and A. Hopkins. 1986. "Being Epileptic: Coming to Terms with Stigma." *Sociology of Health and Illness* 8:26–43.

Scanzoni, J. 1965. "A Note on the Sufficiency of Wife Responses in Family Research." *Pacific Sociological Review* 80:109–115.

Schenk, J., H. Pfrang, and A. Rausche. 1983. "Personality Traits Versus the Quality of the Marital Relationship as the Determinant of Marital Sexuality." *Archives of Sexual Behavior* 12:31–42.

Schneider, D. 1968. *American Kinship*. Englewood Cliffs, N.J.: Prentice-Hall.

Schneider, J. W., and P. Conrad. 1983. *Having Epilepsy*. Philadelphia: Temple University Press.

Science Digest. 1956. "Medical Shopping Decried in Sterility." *Science Digest* 39(5):50.

Scott, R. 1978. *The Making of Blind Men*. New York: Russell Sage.

Scritchfield, S. A. 1989. "The Social Construction of Infertility: From Private Matter to Social Concern." In *Images of Issues: Typifying Contemporary Social Problems*, ed. J. Best, 99–114. New York: Aldine de Gruyter.

Scully, D. 1980. *Men Who Control Women's Health*. Boston: Houghton Mifflin.

Shapiro, C. H. 1988. *Infertility and Pregnancy Loss: A Guide for Helping Professionals*. San Francisco: Jossey-Bass.

Sherman, E., and G. J. Annas. 1986. "Social Policy Considerations in Noncoital Reproduction." *Journal of the American Medical Association* 255:62–68.

Shields, S. A. 1987. "Women, Men, and the Dilemma of Emotion." *Review of Personality and Social Psychology* 7:229–250.

Shields, S. A., and B. Koster. 1989. "Emotional Stereotyping of Parents in Childbearing Manuals, 1915–1980." *Social Psychology Quarterly* 52:44–55.

Shimanoff, S. B. 1983. "The Role of Gender in Linguistic Reference to Emotive States." *Communication Quarterly* 31:174–179.

_____. 1985. "Rules Governing the Verbal Expression of Emotions between Married Couples." *Western Journal of Speech Communication* 49:147–165.

Shostak, A. 1969. *Blue-Collar Life*. New York: Random House.

References

Silva, A. 1962. *A civilzacao indigeno do Uaupés*. Sao Paulo: Centro de Pesquisas de Iauareté.

Simons, H. F. 1984. "Infertility: Implications for Policy Formation." In *Infertility: Medical, Emotional, and Social Considerations*, ed. M. D. Mazor and H. F. Simons, 61–70. New York: Human Sciences Press.

———. 1988. "Resolve Inc.: Advocacy within a Mutual Support Organization." Ph.D. diss., Brandeis University.

Smith, M. G. 1959. *The Economy of Hausa Communities of Zaria*. Colonial Office Research Studies. London: H. M. Stationery Office.

Snarey, J., L. Son, V. S. Kuehne, S. Hauser, and G. Vaillant. 1987. "The Role of Parenting in Men's Psychosocial Development: A Longitudinal Study of Early Adulthood, Infertility and Midlife Generativity." *Developmental Psychology* 23:593–603.

Solomon, A. 1988. "Integrating Infertility Crisis Counseling into Feminist Practice." *Reproductive and Genetic Engineering* 1:41–49.

Sorenson, J. L. 1976. "Toward a Characterization of Mormon Personality." *Committee on Mormon Society and Culture Newsletter* 2:2–8.

Spallone, P., and D. L. Steinberg, eds. 1987. *Made to Order: The Myth of Reproductive and Genetic Progress*. Oxford: Pergamon.

Spitze, G., and J. Huber. 1982. "Accuracy of Wife's Perception of Husband's Attitude toward Her Employment." *Journal of Marriage and the Family* 44:477–481.

Stack, C. 1974. *All Our Kin: Strategies for Survival in a Black Community*. New York: Harper & Row.

Stage, S. 1979. *Female Complaints: Lydia Pinkham and the Business of Women's Medicine*. New York: Norton.

Stamell, M. 1983. "Infertility: Fighting Back." *New York*, March 21, 32.

Stanworth, M., ed. 1987. *Reproductive Technologies: Gender, Motherhood, and Medicine*. Minneapolis: University of Minnesota Press.

Starr, P. 1982. *The Social Transformation of American Medicine*. New York: Basic Books.

Stein, H. F. 1989. *American Medicine as Culture*. Boulder, Colo.: Westview.

Stephanides, C. S. 1941. "A Sociological Sketch of the Village of Megala Vrisi, Macedonia, Greece." Masters Thesis, Cornell University.

Strauss, A., J. Corbin, S. Faberhaugh, B. G. Glaser, D. Maines, B. Suczek, and C. L. Wiener. 1984. *Chronic Illness and the Quality of Life*. 2d ed. St. Louis: Mosby.

Sturgis, S. H. 1957. "Higher Education, Uterine Fluid, and Sterility." *Fertility and Sterility* 8:1–11.

Summey, P., and M. Hurst. 1986. "Ob/Gyn on the Rise: The Evolution of

References

Professional Ideology in the Twentieth Century-Part I." *Women and Health* 11:133–145.

Sung, L. 1975. "Inheritance and Kinship in Northern Taiwan." Ph.D. diss., Stanford University.

Swain, S. 1989. "Covert Intimacy: Closeness in Men's Friendships." In *Gender in Intimate Relationships*, ed. B. J. Risman and P. Schwartz, 71–86. Belmont, Calif.: Wadsworth.

Syme, S. L., and L. F. Berkman. 1976. "Social Class, Susceptibility, and Sickness." *American Journal of Epidemiology* 104:1–8.

Talayevsa, D. C. 1942. *Sun Chief: The Autobiography of a Hopi Indian*, ed. L. W. Simmons. New Haven: Yale University Press.

Talbert, L. M. 1985. "The Arithmetic of Infertility Therapy." In *Infertility: A Practical Guide for the Physician*, ed. M. G. Hammond and L. M. Talbert, 9–14. Oradell, N.J.: Medical Economics Books.

Templeton, A., and G. Penney. 1982. "The Incidence, Characteristics, and Prognosis of Patients Whose Infertility is Unexplained." *Fertility and Sterility* 37:175–182.

Thoits, P. A. 1985. "Self-Labeling Processes in Mental Illness: The Role of Emotional Deviance." *American Journal of Sociology* 91:221–249.

Thomas, A. K., and M. S. Forest. 1980. "Infertility—A Review of 291 Infertile Couples Over 8 Years." *Fertility and Sterility* 34:106–111.

Thompson, L. 1940. *Southern Lau, Fiji: An Ethnography.*" Bulletin 162. Honolulu: Bernice P. Bishop Museum.

Thompson, L., and A. J. Walker. 1989. "Gender in Families: Women and Men in Marriage, Work, and Parenthood." *Journal of Marriage and the Family* 51:845–871.

Tilt, E. J. 1881. *A Handbook of Uterine Therapeutics and of Diseases of Women.* 4th ed. New York: William Wood.

Todd, A. D. 1982. "The Medicalization of Reproduction." Ph.D. diss., University of California, San Diego.

———. 1989. *Intimate Adversaries: Cultural Conflicts between Doctors and Women Patients.* Philadelphia: University of Pennsylvania Press.

Tschopik, H., Jr. 1951. "The Aymara of Chucuito, Peru: Magic." *Anthropological Papers of the American Museum of Natural History* 44:133–308.

Turner, R. H. 1971. "Deviance Avowal As Neutralization of Commitment." *Social Problems* 19:308–321.

Turner, V. W. 1966. *The Ritual Process: Structure and Anti-Structure.* Ithaca: Cornell University Press.

———. 1967. *The Forest of Symbols: Aspects of Ndembu Ritual.* Ithaca: Cornell University Press.

References

———. 1968. *The Drums of Affliction: A Study of Religious Processes Among the Ndembu of Zambia*. Oxford: Clarendon Press.

———. 1969. *The Ritual Process: Structure and Antistructure*. Ithaca: Cornell University Press.

———. 1975. *Revelation and Divination in Ndembu Ritual*. Ithaca: Cornell University Press.

Tyack, D. 1974. *The One Best System: A History of American Urban Education*. Cambridge: Harvard University Press.

U.S. Bureau of the Census. 1975. *Historical Statistics of the United States: Colonial Times to 1970, Part I*. Washington, D.C.: U.S. Government Printing Office.

———. 1989. *Statistical Abstract of the United States: 1989*. 19th ed. Washington, D.C.: U.S. Government Printing Office.

U.S. Congress, Office of Technology Assessment. 1988. *Infertility: Medical and Social Choices*. Washington, D.C.: U.S. Government Printing Office.

Ubell, E. 1990. "You Don't Have to Be Childless." *Parade*, Jan. 14, 14–15.

Udry, J. R. 1974. *The Social Context of Marriage*. Philadelphia: Lippincott.

Van Es, J. C., and P. Shingi. 1972. "Response Consistency of Husband and Wife for Selected Attitudinal Items." *Journal of Marriage and the Family* 34:741–749.

Van Keep, P. A., and H. Schmidt-Elmendorf. 1975. "Involuntary Childlessness." *Journal of Biosocial Science* 7:37–48.

Veevers, J. 1979. "Voluntary Childlessness: A Review of Issues and Evidence." *Marriage and Family Review* 2:1–26.

———. 1980. *Childless by Choice*. Toronto: Butterworths.

Verkauf, B. 1983. "The Incidence and Outcome of Single-Factor, Multifactorial, and Unexplained Infertility." *American Journal of Obstetrics and Gynecology* 147:175–181.

Villa Rojas, A. 1969. "The Tzeltal." In *Handbook of Middle American Indians*, vol. 7, 195–225. Austin: University of Texas Press.

Waitzkin, H. B. 1983. *The Second Sickness: Contradictions of Capitalist Health Care*. New York: Free Press.

Waitzkin, H. B., and B. Waterman. 1974. *The Exploitation of Illness in Capitalist Society*. Indianapolis: Bobbs-Merrill.

Walker, H. E. 1978. "Sexual Problems and Infertility." *Psychosomatics* 19:477–484.

Wallin, P., and A. L. Clark. 1964. "Religiosity, Sexual Gratification, and Marital Satisfaction in the Middle Years of Marriage." *Social Forces* 42:303–309.

Walters, L. 1979. "Human *In Vitro* Fertilization: A Review of the Ethical Literature." *Hastings Center Report* 1(4):23–43.

Weber, M. 1963. *The Sociology of Religion*. Boston: Beacon.

Weiss, L., and M. F. Lowenthal. 1975. "Life-course Perspective on Friendship." In

Four Stages of Life, ed. M. F. Lowenthal, M. Thurnher, and D. Chiriboga, 48–61. San Francisco: Jossey-Bass.

Wertz, R., and D. C. Wertz. 1977. *Lying-In: History of Childbirth in America*. New York: Free Press.

West, C. 1984. *Routine Complications: Troubles with Talk Between Doctors and Patients*. Bloomington: Indiana University Press.

Wikler, N. J. 1986. "Society's Response to the New Reproductive Technologies: The Feminist Perspectives." *Southern California Law Review* 59:1043–1057.

Wilkening, E. A., and D. E. Morrison. 1963. "A Comparison of Husband and Wife Responses Concerning Who Makes Farm and Home Decisions." *Journal of Marriage and the Family* 25:349–351.

Wilkie, J. R. 1981. "The Trend Toward Delayed Parenthood." *Journal of Marriage and the Family* 43:583–591.

Williams, G. 1984. "The Genesis of Chronic Illness: Narrative Reconstruction." *Sociology of Health and Illness* 6:175–200.

Williams, L. S. 1988. "It's Going to Work for Me: Responses to Failures of IVF." *Birth* 15:153–156.

Wills, T. A., R. L. Weiss, and G. R. Patterson, 1974. "A Behavioral Analysis of the Determinants of Marital Satisfaction." *Journal of Consulting and Clinical Psychology* 42:802–811.

Wolf, A. P., and C. Huang. 1980. *Marriage and Adoption in China, 1845–1945*. Stanford: Stanford University Press.

Wolf, M. 1972. *Women and the Family in Rural Taiwan*. Stanford: Stanford University Press.

Woollett, A. 1985. "Childlessness: Strategies for Coping with Infertility." *International Journal of Behavioral Development* 8:473–482.

Wright, W. 1982. *The Social Logic of Health*. New Brunswick, N.J.: Rutgers University Press.

Zborowski, M., and E. Herzog. 1952. *Life is With People: The Jewish Little-town of Eastern Europe*. New York: International Universities Press.

Zelizer, V. A. 1985. *Pricing the Priceless Child*. New York: Basic Books.

Zola, I. K. 1972. "Medicine as An Institution of Social Control." *Sociological Review* 20:487–504.

———. 1983. *Socio-medical Inquiries: Recollections, Reflections and Reconsiderations*. Philadelphia: Temple University Press.

INDEX

accouchers, 38

adoption: crosscultural aspects of, 8, 10, 40–41, 176–177; decision to pursue, 100–101; decline in availability of, 45; history of, 40–41; interracial, 206–207n7; as option for infertile, 48

age norms: definition of, 51; inability to achieve, 133–134, 175; as internalized by infertile, 64

American College of Obstetricians and Gynecologists, increased membership in, 45

American Fertility Society, increased membership in, 33

American Kinship (Schneider), 52

approach-avoidance script: communicative marriage and, 106; infertility and, 113

artificial insemination: cyclical nature of, 45–46; widespread use of, 42; women focus of treatment in, 66

artificial insemination by donor (AID): reactions to, 94; surrogate motherhood and, 210n3; use of, 31, 69–70

artificial insemination by husband (AIH), use of, 31

basal body temperature (BBT): description of, 29; intrusive nature of, 49, 65–66, 123; use of, in scheduling intercourse, 198n67

Bell, Susan, 41

Bellah, Robert, et al., *Habits of the Heart*, 15

Benedek, Therese, 42

Berger, Peter, *The Sacred Canopy*, 15

Berk, A., 205n10

Bernard, Jessie, 107; *The Future of Marriage*, 18

Bernstein, J., 200–201n15

biographical disruption, 102, 153, 159

blaming the victim. *See* victim, blaming of

blood relationships, importance of, 8, 187–188

Blumstein, Philip, 119–120, 125

body as machine, 53, 74

body failure, 53, 65, 199–200n11

Bohannon, Laura, 8

Bohannon, Paul, 8

Borg, Susan, 69, 102

Borkman, Thomasina, 147

Bury, Michael, 102

Caesarean section, as cause of infertility, 43

Cancian, Francesca, 64, 106

cervical mucus, antibodies in, 31

Charmaz, Kathy, 200n13

childbearing, delayed, effect on infertility rate, 43

childbirth, industrialization of, 36–37

childlessness: as deviant, 51; as option for infertile, 48; rate of, 135; nineteenth century, 40–41

childlessness, voluntary: history of, 135–136; imputed to infertile, 132, 134, 138–139; industrialization and, 135; reproductive impairment and, 6–7

children, value of, 40–41, 66–69, 135, 201n29

chronic illness: infertility as, 48, 102–103; stigma of, 126, 132; theodicy construction and, 172

Clarke, Adele, 37–38

clomiphene citrate: cyclical nature of, 45–46; ovulatory problems and, 30, 42

Collins, John A., 32

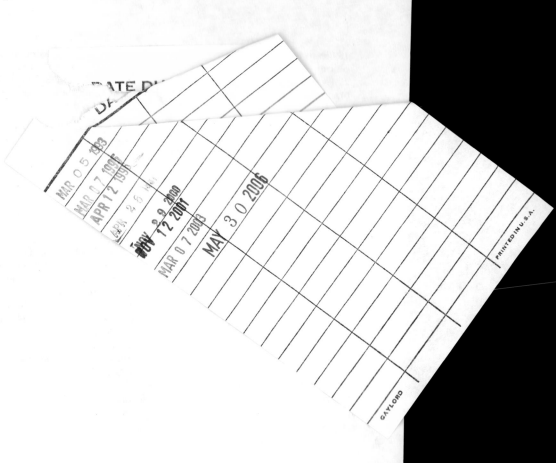